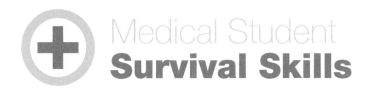

Medical Student
Survival Skills

Procedural Skills

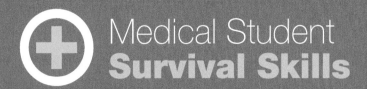

Medical Student
Survival Skills

Procedural Skills

Philip Jevon RN BSc(Hons) PGCE
Academy Manager/Tutor
Walsall Teaching Academy, Manor Hospital, Walsall, UK

Ruchi Joshi FRCS
Clinical Director for Emergency and Acute Medicine
Walsall Healthcare NHS Trust, Manor Hospital, Walsall, UK

Consulting Editors

Jonathan Pepper BMedSci BM BS FRCOG MD FAcadMEd
Consultant Obstetrics and Gynaecology, Head of Academy
Walsall Healthcare NHS Trust, Manor Hospital, Walsall, UK

Jamie Coleman MBChB MD MA(Med Ed) FRCP FBPhS
Professor in Clinical Pharmacology and Medical Education / MBChB Deputy
  Programme Director
School of Medicine, University of Birmingham, Birmingham, UK

WILEY Blackwell

This edition first published 2020
© 2020 by John Wiley & Sons Ltd

The right of Philip Jevon and Ruchi Joshi to be identified as the authors in this work has been asserted in accordance with law.

Registered Office(s)
John Wiley & Sons, Inc., 111 River Street, Hoboken, NJ 07030, USA
John Wiley & Sons Ltd, The Atrium, Southern Gate, Chichester, West Sussex, PO19 8SQ, UK

Editorial Office
9600 Garsington Road, Oxford, OX4 2DQ, UK

For details of our global editorial offices, customer services, and more information about Wiley products visit us at www.wiley.com.

Wiley also publishes its books in a variety of electronic formats and by print-on-demand. Some content that appears in standard print versions of this book may not be available in other formats.

Library of Congress Cataloging-in-Publication Data
Names: Jevon, Philip, author. | Joshi, Ruchi, author.
Title: Medical student survival skills. Procedural skills / Philip Jevon, Ruchi Joshi.
Other titles: Procedural skills
Description: Hoboken, NJ : Wiley-Blackwell, 2020. | Includes index. |
Identifiers: LCCN 2018060342 (print) | LCCN 2018061659 (ebook) | ISBN 9781118870563
  (Adobe PDF) | ISBN 9781118870549 (ePub) | ISBN 9781118870570 (pbk.)
Subjects: | MESH: Clinical Medicine | Clinical Competence | Handbook
Classification: LCC RC46 (ebook) | LCC RC46 (print) | NLM WB 39 | DDC 616–dc23
LC record available at https://lccn.loc.gov/2018060342

Cover Design: Wiley
Cover Image: © WonderfulPixel/Shutterstock

Set in 9.25/12.5pt Helvetica Neue by SPi Global, Pondicherry, India

Printed in Great Britain by TJ International Ltd, Padstow, Cornwall

10 9 8 7 6 5 4 3 2 1

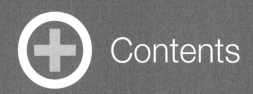

Contents

About the companion website vii

About the companion website

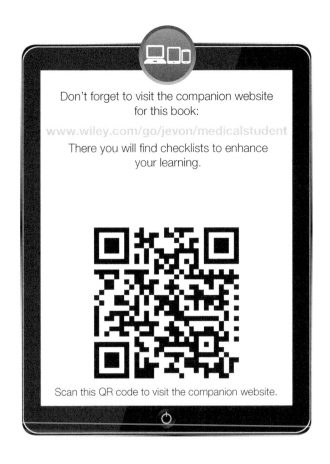

Don't forget to visit the companion website for this book:

www.wiley.com/go/jevon/medicalstudent

There you will find checklists to enhance your learning.

Scan this QR code to visit the companion website.

1 Measuring body temperature

Introduction

- Normal body temperature ranges between 35.8 °C and 37.2 °C (depending on circadian variation and from which part of the body it is measured)
- Core temperature represents the balance between the heat generated by body tissues during metabolic activity, especially of the liver and muscles, and heat lost during various mechanisms
- Taken orally, temperature has been found to be 0.5–1 °C lower than when measured from the rectum
- The most widely used device to measure temperature is the infrared tympanic thermometer (Figure 1.1). This is inserted into the external acoustic meatus and measures the infrared radiation emitted from the tympanic membrane
- Temperature is regulated by the thermoregulatory centre in the hypothalamus through various physiological mechanisms, e.g. sweating, dilation/constriction of peripheral blood vessels and shivering

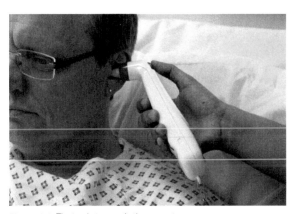

Figure 1.1 Electronic tympanic thermometer.

Medical Student Survival Skills: Procedural Skills, First Edition. Philip Jevon and Ruchi Joshi.
© 2020 John Wiley & Sons Ltd. Published 2020 by John Wiley & Sons Ltd.
Companion website: www.wiley.com/go/jevon/medicalstudent

Indications

- Acute illness – part of the ABCDE approach
- Routine observations

Methods for measuring body temperature

- Tympanic thermometer (most commonly used method)
- Rectal thermometer (particularly in hypothermia)
- Oesophageal/nasopharangeal probes
- Bladder probe
- Pulmonary artery catheter

NB Important definitions:
- *Hypothermia*: <35 °C
- *Hyperthemia*: >37.5 °C

Procedure using an electronic tympanic thermometer

- Assemble equipment: electronic tympanic thermometer, new hygiene probe, and waste bag
- Identify correct patient
- Introduce yourself to the patient
- Explain procedure to the patient and gain consent
- Ascertain which ear was used for previous readings
- Wash hands
- Turn on electronic thermometer and attach new hygienic probe cover following manufacturer's recommendations
- Gently pull back the pinna upwards and backwards and insert the thermometer in the external acoustic meatus (Figure 1.2)
- Press the button on the device to measure the temperature and a reading should appear
- Remove the thermometer from the ear canal and then dispose of the hygiene probe into the waste bag
- Wash hands
- Document information on temperature chart of correctly identified patient including time and date taken

- Clear away equipment and ensure that the electronic tympanic thermometer is stored following the manufacturer's guidelines

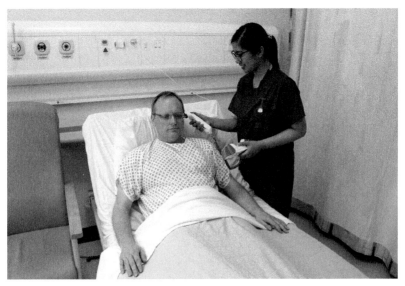

Figure 1.2 Inserting an electronic tympanic thermometer.

OSCE Key Learning Points

Good practice

- ✔ Wash and dry hands
- ✔ Use the same ear for consecutive measurements
- ✔ Install a new disposable probe cover for each measurement
- ✔ Ensure thermometer probe is positioned snugly in the external auditory meatus
- ✔ Aim thermometer towards the tympanic membrane
- ✔ Measure the patient's temperature following manufacturer's instructions
- ✔ Consider the temperature reading alongside other systemic observations and overall condition of the patient
- ✔ Store the thermometer following manufacturer's instructions

Mechanisms of heat loss

- *Radiation*: flow of heat from a higher temperature (the body) to a lower temperature (environment surrounding the body)
- *Convection*: heat transfer by flow or movement of air
- *Conduction*: heat transfer due to direct contact with cooler surfaces
- *Evaporation*: perspiration, respiration, and breaks in skin integrity

Factors that can cause a fluctuation in body temperature

- The body's *circadian rhythms*: temperature is higher in the evening than the morning; the difference can be as much as 1.5 °C. If temperature is being recorded every 4–6 hours, the optimum time for detecting a pyrexia is probably between 7 and 8 p.m.
- *Ovulation*
- *Exercise* and *eating* can cause a rise in temperature
- *Old age*: there is an increased sensitivity to cold and there is generally a lower body temperature
- *Illness*, e.g. sepsis

NB The tympanic membrane shares the same carotid blood supply as the hypothalamus; measurement of the tympanic membrane temperature therefore reflects core temperature.

Common misinterpretations and pitfalls

Care should be taken when using the tympanic thermometer as poor technique can render the measurement inaccurate. Temperature differences between the opening of the ear canal and the tympanic membrane can be as much as 2.8 °C.

NB Ear canal size, wax, operator technique, and the patient's position can affect the accuracy of the measurements.

Causes of pyrexia

- Infection
- Hyperthyroidism
- Malignancy
- Drug allergy
- Surgery – tissue damage
- Damage to the central nervous system
- Allergic reaction to blood transfusion
- Heat stroke

 Common misinterpretations and pitfalls

- Pyrexia in response to infection is a protective mechanism. It inhibits bacterial and viral growth, promotes immunity and phagocytosis, and through hypermetabolism promotes tissue repair. Mild pyrexia is generally not treated
- Care should be taken to ensure the same method/site for recording temperature is used to help ensure the recordings are reliable

2 Measuring pulse and blood pressure

Assessment of pulse

- Assess the patient's radial pulse
- Hold the patient's right hand and palpate the radial pulse using the tips of the index and middle fingers (the pulse can be felt on the radial aspect of the flexor surface of the forearm, a few centimetres proximal to the wrist)
- Count the rate of the pulse, e.g. using a watch with a second hand, count the number of beats in 30 seconds and multiply this by 2; care should be taken if the pulse is irregular. A normal pulse rate is considered to be between 60 and 100 min^{-1}, a tachycardia is a pulse rate > 100 min^{-1} and a bradycardia is a pulse rate < 60 min^{-1}
- Assess the rhythm of the pulse; is it regular or irregular (the rate usually quickens during inspiration – sinus arrhythmia). An irregular pulse is usually either due to ectopic beats or atrial fibrillation
- Palpate both radial pulses together and compare: differences between the two may indicate acute aortic dissection or proximal arterial disease
- Compare the apex beat with the radial pulse and check for a pulse deficit (in atrial fibrillation the heart rate is sometimes faster than the pulse, the difference being termed *pulse deficit*)
- Assess the volume of the pulse; a rapid, weak, thready pulse is a characteristic sign of shock. A full bounding or throbbing pulse may be indicative of anaemia, heart block, heart failure, or the early stages of septic shock
- Check for a collapsing pulse (sign of aortic regurgitation): using the palm of the left hand, grasp the patient's right distal forearm and elevate; a vibrating pulse felt in the fingers indicates a collapsing pulse
- Compare the central (femoral or carotid) and distal (radial) pulses: a discrepancy in the volume between them could be due to a fall in cardiac output (and also cold ambient temperature)

Medical Student Survival Skills: Procedural Skills, First Edition. Philip Jevon and Ruchi Joshi.
© 2020 John Wiley & Sons Ltd. Published 2020 by John Wiley & Sons Ltd.
Companion website: www.wiley.com/go/jevon/medicalstudent

Assessment of perfusion: Capillary refill time

Decreased skin perfusion is often characterised by cool peripheries, skin mottling, pallor, cyanosis, and delayed capillary refill (>2 seconds). The following procedure is suggested for the assessment of capillary refill:

- Explain the procedure to the patient
- Elevate the extremity, e.g. digit, slightly higher than the level of the heart (this will ensure the assessment of arteriolar capillary and not venous stasis refill)
- Blanch the digit for 5 seconds and then release. A sluggish (delayed) capillary refill (>2 seconds) may be caused by circulatory shock, pyrexia, or a cold ambient temperature

Non-Invasive blood pressure measurement

Of all the measurements routinely undertaken in clinical practice, the recording of blood pressure is potentially the most unreliably and incorrectly performed measurement. It is essential that blood pressure recordings are accurate and reliable: good practice can significantly reduce measurement errors and help ensure that the blood pressure recording obtained is accurate and reliable.

Approximately 40% of adults in England and Wales have hypertension (this percentage increases with age) – a significant risk factor for stroke, chronic renal failure, and coronary heart disease.

Systolic and diastolic blood pressure

- *Systolic blood pressure*: peak blood pressure in the artery following ventricular systole (contraction)
- *Diastolic blood pressure*: level to which the arterial blood pressure falls during ventricular diastole (relaxation)

Korotkoff's sounds

Five different sound phases known as Korotkoff's sounds (Korotkoff, a Russian surgeon, first described the auscultation method of measuring blood pressure in 1905) can be heard as the blood pressure cuff is slowly released:

- Phase 1: a thud
- Phase 2: a blowing or swishing noise
- Phase 3: a softer thud than in phase 1
- Phase 4: a disappearing blowing noise
- Phase 5: silence

Practically, the systolic reading is when the Korotkoff sounds are first heard and the diastolic reading is when the sounds disappear.

Which arm?

The blood pressure should initially be measured in both arms and the arm with the higher readings should be used for subsequent measurements. Although a difference in blood pressure measurements between the arms can be expected in 20% of patients, if this difference is >20 mmHg for systolic or >10 mmHg for diastolic on three consecutive readings, further investigation will probably be indicated.

Procedure for manual measurement of blood pressure

The traditional manual blood pressure device using auscultation is still a very popular, and when used correctly, reliable method of recording blood pressure. The following procedure for its use is recommended.

- Ideally ensure that the patient has been sitting or lying down for at least 5 minutes and is comfortably relaxed
- Check the equipment, ensuring it is in good working order
- Explain the procedure to the patient and obtain their consent
- Ask the patient to remove any tight clothing from around the arm
- Ensure the patient's arm is supported at the level of the heart. If the arm is unsupported, the blood pressure is likely to be erroneously increased due to muscle contraction in the arm. If the arm is higher than the level of the heart, this can lead to an underestimation of the diastolic pressure by as much as 10 mmHg
- Select an appropriately sized cuff: the bladder of the cuff should encircle at least 80% of the arm but no more than 100%
- Place the cuff snugly onto the patient's arm, with the centre of the bladder over the brachial artery – most cuffs have a 'brachial artery indicator', an arrow which should be aligned with the brachial artery
- Position the sphygmomanometer near to the patient. It should be vertical and at the nurse's eye level
- Ask the patient to refrain from talking or eating during the procedure as this can result in an inaccurate, higher blood pressure
- Estimate the systolic pressure: palpate the brachial artery, inflate the cuff, and note the reading when the brachial pulse disappears. Then deflate the cuff

- Inflate the cuff to 30 mmHg above the estimated systolic level that was required to occlude the brachial pulse. Approximately 5% of the population has an auscultatory gap; this is when Korotkoff's sounds disappear just below the systolic pressure and reappear above the diastolic pressure. Estimating the systolic pressure will help ensure that the cuff is sufficiently inflated to record an accurate systolic pressure
- Palpate the brachial artery
- Place the diaphragm of the stethoscope gently over the brachial artery. Avoid applying excessive pressure on the diaphragm and do not tuck the diaphragm under the edge of the cuff because either of these actions could partially occlude the brachial artery, delaying the occurrence of the Korotoff sounds
- Open the valve and slowly deflate the cuff at a rate of 2–3 mm s^{-1}, recording when the Korotkoff sounds first appear (systolic) and disappear (diastolic)
- Document the systolic and diastolic blood pressure readings on the patient's observation chart following local protocols. Compare with previous readings and inform the nurse in charge/medical team as appropriate

 Common misinterpretations and pitfalls

Errors in blood pressure measurement can occur for several reasons including:

- Defective equipment, e.g. leaky tubing or a faulty valve
- Failure to ensure the mercury column reads 0 mmHg at rest
- Too rapid deflation of the cuff
- Use of incorrectly sized cuff: if it is too small the blood pressure will be overestimated and if it is too big the blood pressure will be underestimated
- Cuff not at the same level as the heart
- Failure to observe the mercury level properly – the top of the mercury column should be at eye level
- Poor technique (e.g. failing to note when the sounds disappear)
- Digit preference, rounding the reading up to the nearest 5 or 10 mmHg
- Observer bias, e.g. expecting a young patient's blood pressure to be normal

Automated blood pressure devices

When automated blood pressure devices were first manufactured, their accuracy and reliability was questioned. However, improved technology has led to the development of more accurate and reliable devices, some of which have been tested and approved for use by the British Hypertensive Society.

Most automated devices measure blood pressure using one of the following techniques:

- Oscillometry to detect arterial blood flow (most commonly used device)
- A microphone to detect the Korotkoff sounds
- Ultrasound to detect arterial blood flow

Procedure for automated measurement of blood pressure

The principles for the accurate measurement of blood pressure using an automated electronic device are similar to those of the manual recording of blood pressure using a sphygmomanometer in respect of patient preparation, patient position, and cuff choice/placement. However, when using an automated electronic device, it is important to be familiar with its working and to follow the manufacturer's recommendations when using it.

③ Transcutaneous monitoring of oxygen saturations

Introduction

- Transcutaneous monitoring of oxygen saturations is also known as pulse oximetry
- The procedure involves a quick, cheap, and non-invasive bedside monitor which can play a vital role in the assessment of hypoxaemia
- It is a method of providing an objective and continuous recording of arterial blood oxygen saturation
- The pulse oximeter probe emits light from light emitting diodes (LEDs) through the tissue
- The pulse oximeter measures oxygen saturation by calculating the ratio of light that passes through the tissue to that which does not
- This is accurate to ± 2% above a saturation of 90%

Indications

Pulse oximetry can be useful as part of the assessment of:
- Monitoring of acutely ill patients
- Targeted oxygen therapy
- Asthma/chronic obstructive pulmonary disease (COPD)
- Diagnosis of sleep apnoea
- Confused patients
- Monitoring during general anaesthesia

NB Central cyanosis is also a sign of hypoxaemia but this only manifests when saturations are as low as 75–80%.

Medical Student Survival Skills: Procedural Skills, First Edition. Philip Jevon and Ruchi Joshi.
© 2020 John Wiley & Sons Ltd. Published 2020 by John Wiley & Sons Ltd.
Companion website: www.wiley.com/go/jevon/medicalstudent

Cautions

Anything that interferes with the transmission of light through the tissue may affect oxygen saturation readings. Other errors can be caused by:

- Nail varnish
- Reduced pulse volume (low cardiac output, hypotension, hypothermia)
- Other haemoglobins (such as carbon monoxide, sickle cells, or foetal haemoglobin)
- Motion artefact

 NB Ensure appropriately sized probes are used for infants and children.

Contraindications

- There are no contraindications

Equipment

- Pulse oximeter

Procedure for transcutaneous monitoring of oxygen saturations

Pre-procedure

- Ensure pulse oximeter is working (check battery)
- Identify correct patient
- Explain procedure to the patient
- Wash hands

Procedure

- Place pulse oximeter onto patient's finger, ensuring the digit is fully inserted into the probe
- Rest the hand with the probe on the chest at the level of the heart. This also reduces motion artefact
- Readings should be taken for 2–5 minutes or it can be left on for continuous monitoring

Post-procedure

- Remove pulse oximeter from the patient's finger
- Manage the patient according to pulse oximetry findings as well as clinical findings
  - Normal oxygen saturations: 94% or above
  - In COPD patients, saturations between 88% and 92% may be acceptable

OSCE Key Learning Points

If unable to obtain a pulse oximeter reading

✔ Rub skin to warm up

✔ Try a different site (different finger or ear lobe)

✔ Use topical vasodilator

✔ Try different machine

✔ Reassess patient! – they may be very hypoxic, hypotensive, or peripherally shut down

Complications

- Prolonged pulse oximetry may cause irritation or breakdown of the tissue at the probe site

Common misinterpretations and pitfalls

- The oxyhaemoglobin dissociation curve demonstrates the relationship between oxygen saturation and PaO_2 (oxygen partial pressure)
- The shape of the curve means that below saturations of ~90%, PaO_2 has dropped by about 50% of its norm – early hypoxaemia may be masked!
- Oxygen saturations can be normal even if the patient is acutely ill

4 Peak expiratory flow

Introduction

- Peak expiratory flow (PEF) can be defined as the maximum flow achieved on forced expiration from a position of full inspiration
- A simple method of measuring the degree of airway obstruction, it helps to detect and monitor moderate and severe respiratory disease
- It is mainly used in the diagnosis and monitoring of asthma, particularly when assessing the severity of an asthma attack and monitoring the response to therapy

Peak expiratory flow

- PEF reflects a range of physiological characteristics of the lungs, airways, and neuromuscular characteristics of individuals, including lung elastic recoil, large airway calibre, lung volume, effort, and neuromuscular integrity
- The reflection of airway calibre makes the PEF meter suitable for measuring variations in PEF over time to provide support for:
  - Confirmation of the diagnosis of asthma
  - Diagnosis of occupational asthma
  - Monitoring variation in PEF over time
  - Identification of asthma control
  - Use in self-management of asthma by patients via written action plans based on changes in PEF

Indications for recording PEF

- Usually undertaken four times a day, both before and after the administration of bronchodilators

Medical Student Survival Skills: Procedural Skills, First Edition. Philip Jevon and Ruchi Joshi.
© 2020 John Wiley & Sons Ltd. Published 2020 by John Wiley & Sons Ltd.
Companion website: www.wiley.com/go/jevon/medicalstudent

- Normally in asthmatic patients – provides an indicator of how well the patient's asthma is responding to treatment and an aid in measuring the recovery from an asthma attack
- Acute asthma attack – to help determine severity of attack

PEF readings

- Normal range for PEF readings are influenced by age, sex, and height
- Usually higher in men than women and they peak in the 30–40 year age group
- PEF varies throughout the day; often higher in the evenings than in the mornings
- Nunn and Gregg's reference values for normal PEF flow readings are widely accepted
- When assessing the severity of an asthma attack:
  - PEF reading <50% of the reference value indicates severe asthma
  - PEF reading <33% of the reference value indicates life-threatening asthma

Procedure

- Wash and dry hands
- Assemble the necessary equipment: PEF meter, a clean mouth piece, and the patient's observation chart/PEF diary
- Explain the procedure to the patient and obtain their consent
- Set the pointer on the peak flow meter scale to zero (Figure 4.1)
- Ask the patient to adopt a comfortable position, either sitting or standing. It is important to ensure that the same position is used
- Ask the patient to take a deep breath in through the mouth to full inspiration
- Holding the PEF meter horizontally, ask the patient to place their lips and teeth around the mouth piece, ensuring a good seal
- Ask the patient to breathe out as hard and as fast as possible into the PEF meter (Figure 4.2)
- Note the reading on the PEF meter and then return the pointer to zero
- Ask the patient to repeat the procedure twice; after each time note the reading on the PEF meter scale and return the pointer on the scale to zero
- Document the highest of the three readings following local protocols. Inform the nurse in charge if the PEF reading is abnormal
- Dispose of the mouth piece

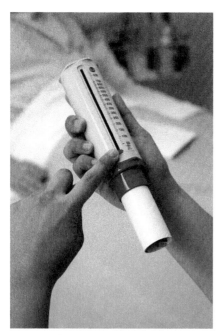

Figure 4.1 Set the pointer on the peak flow meter scale to zero.

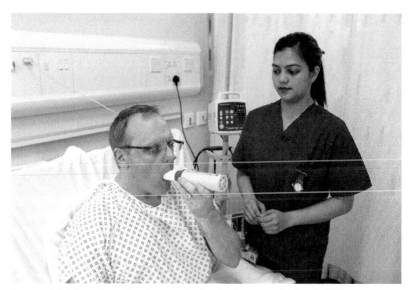

Figure 4.2 Ask the patient to breathe out as hard and as fast as possible into the PEF meter.

Common misinterpretations and pitfalls

Potential unreliable readings:
- Failing to take a deep breath in
- Incorrect exhaling technique, e.g. 'coughing' or 'spitting' technique
- Blocking the mouth piece with the tongue or teeth
- Lack of an effective seal between the mouth piece and the patient's mouth

(5) Venepuncture

Introduction

- Venepuncture is the introduction of a needle into a vein to obtain a blood sample for haematological, biochemical, or microbiological analysis
- It can be performed with a variety of equipment and blood can be taken from many sites
- Vacutainers are the most commonly used devices (Figure 5.1)
- A needle and syringe can also be used
- Butterfly needles are particularly useful for veins that are smaller in size

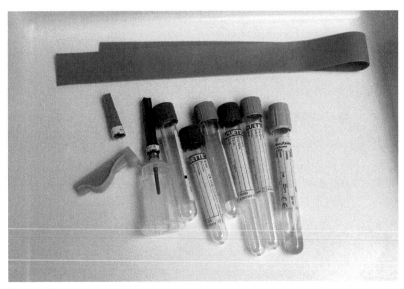

Figure 5.1 Vacutainer device and needle.

Medical Student Survival Skills: Procedural Skills, First Edition. Philip Jevon and Ruchi Joshi.
© 2020 John Wiley & Sons Ltd. Published 2020 by John Wiley & Sons Ltd.
Companion website: www.wiley.com/go/jevon/medicalstudent

Equipment

- Needle
- Vacutainer connection/syringe
- Gloves (non-sterile)
- Alcohol prep pads/ChloraPrep to clean area
- Tourniquet
- Sharps bin
- Apron
- Gauze and tape/plaster
- Blood bottles

Procedure

Pre-procedure

- Prepare equipment
- Identify correct patient
- Explain procedure to the patient and gain their consent
- Wash hands and don apron
- Allow the patient to get into a comfortable position – e.g. resting their arm on a pillow

Procedure

- Apply tourniquet to identify a suitable vein and palpate it – it should feel 'springy' to touch and be easily compressible (and not have a palpable pulse)
- You can ask the patient to clench/unclench their fist or dangle their arm over the side of the bed to enhance the vein's prominence

 NB Never leave a tourniquet on for more than 90 seconds.

- Remove tourniquet and clean the area with alcohol prep pads/ChloraPrep
- Ensure all equipment is to hand, particularly the sharps bin
- Don non-sterile gloves and reapply tourniquet
- Use your non-dominant hand, hold some gauze in your palm, and apply manual traction to the skin below the vein to immobilise it

- Insert the needle into the vein, in the direction of the vein at an angle of around 30° to the skin's surface, and check for flashback (Figure 5.2)
- If there is no flashback, try moving the needle slightly further in or pulling it back a bit, ensuring you are following the course of the vein
- Once you have obtained sufficient blood, unclip or untie the tourniquet and place your gauze over the needle. Remove the needle and put it straight into the sharps bin

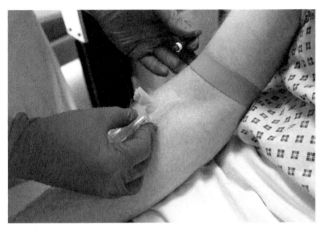

Figure 5.2 Insert the needle into the vein.

NB Always dispose of sharps immediately into the sharps bin to avoid needle-stick injuries.

- Press the gauze firmly onto the puncture site for 2 minutes, check there is no further bleeding, and apply a dressing/plaster
- Make sure blood is in the appropriate bottles, then place in a bag for them to be sent to the lab. Clean equipment tray and dispose of rubbish. Remove gloves and apron and wash hands

Post-procedure
- Ensure that the patient is comfortable
- Ensure that they are no longer having significant bleeding from the venepuncture site

OSCE Key Learning Points

✔ Ensure the procedure is performed as cleanly as possible
✔ Ensure safe use of the tourniquet
✔ Take care when inserting and removing the needle
✔ Ensure safe disposal of sharps

Complications

- Bleeding from venepuncture site
- Infection at site
- Bruising and tenderness at site

Managing blood samples correctly

Introduction

This is an important skill to master and will comprise a large proportion your workload as a foundation doctor.

Indications

- Clinical diagnosis
- Monitoring and assessment of efficacy of treatment

Contraindications

Do not take blood from an arm when:
- The patient has refused
- There is a IV drip running as it will alter results
- The patient has undergone a mastectomy on that side
- They have an arteriovenous (AV) fistula
- The vessel you are palpating has a pulse

Equipment

- Needle
- Barrel/Vacutainer bottles – or equivalent collection system
- Tourniquet
- Alcohol swab
- Cotton wool
- Tape

Medical Student Survival Skills: Procedural Skills, First Edition. Philip Jevon and Ruchi Joshi.
© 2020 John Wiley & Sons Ltd. Published 2020 by John Wiley & Sons Ltd.
Companion website: www.wiley.com/go/jevon/medicalstudent

Procedure for venepuncture

Pre-procedure

- Wash your hands and get your equipment ready. Collect all the sample bottles that you will need and do not forget the sharps bin. Gloves are worn for your protection and not the patients
- Introduce yourself and check they are the correct patient by checking their name and their date of birth on their wristband and verbally
- Explain the procedure and why you are doing it, with the risks involved. Consent in this circumstance can be verbal or implied (patient moves arm so that procedure can be performed)
- Check for allergies and anticoagulant medication

Procedure

- Expose the patient's arm and place the tourniquet on it about 2–3 cm above the antecubital fossa (ACF). Look and palpate for a vein. If there is nothing apparent ask the patient to clench and open their fist a few times
- If you really cannot find any veins in the ACF then look elsewhere, for example the back of the hands or even the feet
- When you have found a vein, clean the area with an alcohol wipe or ChloraPrep for 30 seconds and allow to dry
- Anchor the vein just below where you are going to puncture, hold the needle at 20–30° to the arm, and push it into the vein with the bevel upwards. Advance 2–3 mm into the vein; when you are confident that you are into the vein, if you are using Vacutainer, then attach the required blood bottles and allow them to fill
- Remove the tourniquet when you have all the samples you require and cover the entry site with cotton wool, applying firm pressure

Post-procedure

- Dispose of needles straight into the sharps bin
- Label up your blood samples, double checking for accuracy
- Clean up after yourself, wash your hands, and thank the patient

Complications

Complications are rare when the procedure is performed properly, but include:

- Infection
- Pain
- Haematoma/bruising
- Nerve damage

Blood tubes

Colours of blood test tubes and what they do vary between hospitals and different venepuncture systems, so you will have to check locally what colours are used for each sample in your hospital. Table 6.1 gives a summary of what to consider when choosing blood bottles.

Table 6.1 Blood tubes and different tests

Test	Contents of tube	Additional information
Haematology (full blood count [FBC], reticulocytes, haemoglobin [Hb] electrophoresis, sicke cell screen)	Ethylenediamine tetra-acetic acid (EDTA)	Gently mix 1 ml needed
Erythrocyte sedimentation rate (ESR)	EDTA	Gently mix Fill to the line or it will be rejected
Group and save (G&S)	EDTA	4 ml meeded Usually hand written
Clotting (D-dimer, international normalised ratio [INR], activated partial thromboplastin time [APTT], thrombophillia screen)	Sodium citrate	Gently mix Fill to the line or it will be rejected
Biochemistry (urea and electrolytes [U&Es], liver function tests [LFTs], amylase, thyroid function test [TFT], C-reactive protein [CRP], Ca^{2+}, Mg^{2+}, Cl^-, lactate dehydrogenase [LDH], majority of drug levels, tumour markers, beta-human chorionic gonadotrophin [β-HCG])	Glucose separating gel	If possible use green venepuncture needles to avoid haemolysis 1.5 ml needed
Endocrinology tests	Plain or with heparin	Check with lab for specific tests in order to avoid mistakes May need to be taken on ice to lab

Group and save

When taking a sample for G&S for blood transfusion is it important that the sample is *hand written at the patient's bedside*. Although bedside checks are always important is is particularly important to do these checks extremely carefully as the implications of an incorrect sample are severe. If there are any omissions in patient details or illegible writing on the blood bottle, it will almost certainly be rejected by the laboratory. This is not only annoying for the patient who will have to undergo another venepuncture but also wastes your time, and in an emergency situation it can cause unnecessary delays. Therefore, ensure you get it right first time and check, check, CHECK.

NB
- Wear gloves when handling any bodily fluids, it is for your own protection
- Always check patient details carefully to prevent errors
- Dispose of your equipment appropriately

7 Taking blood cultures

Introduction

Blood cultures should be taken from patients with suspected sepsis in order to tailor antimicrobial therapies.

Indications

Blood cultures are taken to confirm suspected bacteraemia. Indications include:

- Core temperature out of normal range (there is no absolute temperature below which blood cultures are not required)
- Focal signs of infection
- Signs of sepsis
- Chills or rigors
- Raised or very low peripheral blood white cell count
- New or worsening confusion

Equipment

- Needle
- Vacutainer connection/syringe
- Gloves (non-sterile)
- Alcohol prep pads/ChloraPrep to clean area
- Tourniquet
- Sharps bin
- Apron
- Gauze and tape/plaster
- Appropriate blood culture bottles (Figure 7.1, Table 7.1)

Medical Student Survival Skills: Procedural Skills, First Edition. Philip Jevon and Ruchi Joshi.
© 2020 John Wiley & Sons Ltd. Published 2020 by John Wiley & Sons Ltd.
Companion website: www.wiley.com/go/jevon/medicalstudent

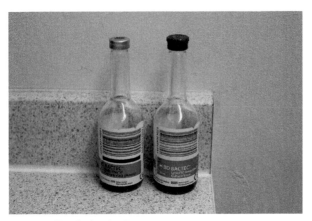

Figure 7.1 Blood culture bottles.

Table 7.1 Blood culture bottle types, associated blood volumes, and indications

Bottle type	Colour	Blood volume	Indication for use
Aerobic	Blue	8–10 ml	All routine blood cultures
Anaerobic	Yellow	5–7 ml	Add one anaerobic bottle to each aerobic bottle in suspected endocarditis and pyrexia of unknown origin (PUO)
Mycobacteria	Red	1–5 ml	Suspected disseminated mycobacterial infection
Paediatric	Pink	1–3 ml	Infants and young children where only small volumes of blood are available

Procedure

Pre-procedure

- Prepare equipment and clean your equipment tray. Remove culture bottle covers and clean the tops with alcohol swab.
- Identify correct patient
- Explain procedure to the patient and gain their consent
- Wash hands and don apron
- Allow the patient to get into a comfortable position – e.g. resting their arm on a pillow

Procedure

- Apply tourniquet to identify a suitable vein and palpate it – it should feel 'springy' to touch and be easily compressible (and not have a palpable pulse)
- You can ask the patient to clench/unclench their fist or dangle their arm over the side of the bed to enhance the vein's prominence

NB Never leave a tourniquet on for more than 90 seconds.

- Remove tourniquet and clean area with alcohol wipes/ChloraPrep
- Ensure all equipment is to hand, particularly the sharps bin
- Don non-sterile gloves and reapply tourniquet. Do not re-palpate the area, it must be sterile
- Use your non-dominant hand, hold some gauze in your palm, and apply manual traction to the skin below the vein to immobilise it
- Insert the needle into the vein, in the direction of the vein at an angle of around 30° to the skin's surface, and check for flashback
- If there is no flashback, try moving needle slightly further in or pulling it back a bit, ensuring you are following the course of the vein
- With a needle and syringe, gently pull back the plunger to obtain blood. With a Vacutainer, attach the culture bottle to its attachment with the needle and remove it when sufficient blood is obtained. Fill the anaerobic culture bottle first

 NB Always fill the anaerobic culture bottle first.

- Once you have obtained sufficient blood, unclip or untie the tourniquet and place your gauze over the needle. Remove the needle and put it straight into the sharps bin

 NB Always dispose of sharps immediately into the sharps bin to avoid needle-stick injuries.

- Press the gauze firmly onto the puncture site for 2 minutes, check there is no further bleeding, and apply a dressing/plaster
- Invert the culture bottles several times to mix and ensure that they are labelled correctly
- Clean equipment tray and dispose of rubbish. Remove gloves and apron and wash hands

Post-procedure

- Ensure that the patient is comfortable and that they are no longer having significant bleeding from the venepuncture site

- Ensure the blood culture bottles are labelled following local policy
- Ensure the blood culture bottles are stored and collected following local policy

OSCE Key Learning Points

✔ Ensure the procedure is performed as cleanly as possible
✔ Ensure safe use of the tourniquet
✔ Take care when inserting and removing the needle
✔ Ensure safe disposal of sharps

Complications

- Bleeding from venepuncture site
- Infection at site
- Bruising and tenderness at site

 NB Blood cultures should be taken before commencing antibiotics. If the patient is already on antibiotics, blood cultures should be taken immediately before the next dose.

 Common misinterpretations and pitfalls

Do not use existing peripheral lines/cannulas or sites immediately above peripheral lines.

8 Measuring capillary blood glucose

Introduction

- Measuring capillary blood glucose (CBG) is a simple and quick investigation
- The sticks used to measure it are commonly known as 'BM sticks'
- Measuring blood glucose levels is useful in patients with diabetes mellitus but is also useful in any unwell patient
- This technique for this procedure is the same as that for measuring capillary ketone levels
- The normal range for CBG is 4–7 mmol l^{-1}

Hypoglycaemia (low blood sugar)

Causes

- Illness – e.g. sepsis, acute liver failure, adrenal/pituitary insufficiency
- Recent physical exertion
- Missed meal/snack
- Not enough carbohydrate-containing food
- Overdosed hypoglycaemic medication or insulin (intentional or unintentional/iatrogenic)
- Acute liver failure
- Alcohol

Symptoms and signs

Symptoms	Signs
Sweating	Pallor
Hunger	Slurred speech/focal neurology
Shaking	Tremor, seizures
Symptoms of infection	Signs of infection
Confusion	Coma

Medical Student Survival Skills: Procedural Skills, First Edition. Philip Jevon and Ruchi Joshi.
© 2020 John Wiley & Sons Ltd. Published 2020 by John Wiley & Sons Ltd.
Companion website: www.wiley.com/go/jevon/medicalstudent

Hyperglycaemia (high blood sugar)

Causes

- Artefact – sugar on skin (e.g. patient just handled a sweet)
- Illness – e.g. sepsis, myocardial infarction, trauma, surgery
- Recent meal/snack
- Missed/underdosed hypoglycaemic medication or insulin
- Medications – e.g. steroids
- New diagnosis of diabetes mellitus

Symptoms and signs

Symptoms	Signs
Nausea	Vomiting
Thirst	Polyuria, urinary frequency
Blurred vision	Delirium
Abdominal pain	Signs of infection
Confusion	
Symptoms of infection	

 NB With any deranged CBG measurement, repeat it – especially if the patient's clinical condition does not match the measurement.

Indications

- Routine monitoring of diabetic patients during an in-patient stay – performed more frequently when a patient is unwell, has unstable CBGs, or is on insulin
- Any patient with symptoms/signs of deranged blood sugar level
- Unwell patients (to exclude deranged blood sugar as a cause or exacerbating factor of their unwell condition)

Equipment

- Disinfectant wipe
- Lancet
- CBG stick
- CBG machine

- Gauze
- Sharps box

Procedure for measurement

Pre-procedure

- Gather equipment
- Identify correct patient
- Confirm reason for CBG measurement
- Explain procedure to patient, e.g. that they will feel a sharp scratch

Procedure

- Remove CBG measuring stick from packet and insert into CBG machine
- Clean patient's finger
- Gently squeeze finger
- Prick skin to draw blood using a lancet or similar device
- Gently squeeze finger to encourage blood to form a drop on the skin
- Collect blood with CBG stick until machine indicates enough has been provided
- Place gauze over skin prick and ask patient to apply gentle pressure
- Read and interpret result

Post-procedure

- Dispose of lancet in sharps bin
- Document result on correct patient's CBG chart
- Inform nursing staff of change in frequency of CBG monitoring if necessary (e.g. if giving insulin to lower CBG), and repeat CBG after 2 hours
- Inform clinical staff of CBG result if appropriate

OSCE Key Learning Points

- Correct technique of obtaining blood for sample
- Correct interpretation of results

 Common misinterpretations and pitfalls

The signs of hypoglycaemia may be mistaken for drunkenness.

9 ECG monitoring

Introduction

- An electrocardiograph is a machine that records the waveforms generated by the heart's electrical activity
- An electrocardiogram (ECG) is a record or display of a person's heartbeat produced by an electrocardiograph
- Bedside ECG monitoring

Indications

- Critical illness
- Acute coronary syndromes
- Cardiac arrhythmias
- History of syncope
- History of palpitations
- During general anaesthetic/surgery

ECG monitoring: Three cable system

- Red ECG cable: below the right clavicle
- Yellow ECG cable: below the left clavicle
- Green ECG cable: left lower thorax/hip region

ECG monitoring: Five cable system

- RA (red ECG cable): below the right clavicle
- LA (yellow ECG cable): below the left clavicle
- RL (black ECG cable): right lower thorax/hip region
- LL (green ECG cable): left lower thorax/hip region
- V (white ECG cable): on the chest in the desired V position, usually V1 (4th intercostal space just right of the sternum)

Medical Student Survival Skills: Procedural Skills, First Edition. Philip Jevon and Ruchi Joshi.
© 2020 John Wiley & Sons Ltd. Published 2020 by John Wiley & Sons Ltd.
Companion website: www.wiley.com/go/jevon/medicalstudent

Procedure

- Explain the procedure to the patient
- Ensure the skin is dry, not greasy; clean with an alcohol swab and/or abrasive pad
- Shave off any dense hair – this is to help ensure better contact and make it less uncomfortable for the patient when the ECG electrodes are removed
- Check the ECG electrodes to ensure they are in date and still moist, not dry
- Remove the protective backing from the ECG electrodes to expose the gel disc
- Place the ECG electrodes on the patient. Using a circular motion, smooth down the adhesive area. Avoid applying pressure on the gel disc itself as this could result in a decrease in electrode conductivity and adherence. The electrodes should lie flat. If the electrodes have an offset connector (to absorb tugs) these should be pointed in the direction of the ECG cables. A standard position for the electrodes is:
  - Red: right shoulder
  - Yellow: left shoulder
  - Green: lower left chest wall
- Correctly attach the ECG cables to the electrodes
- Switch on the cardiac monitor and select the required monitoring ECG lead (usually lead II)
- Ensure the ECG trace displayed is clear. Rectify any difficulties encountered
- Set the alarms within safe parameters following locally agreed protocols and appropriate for the condition of the patient
- Secure the ECG cables, ensuring that they will not tug on the ECG electrodes
- Position the cardiac monitor so it is clearly visible to the nursing staff
- Document in the patient's notes that ECG monitoring has commenced and the ECG rhythm identified
- Monitor the electrode sites regularly for signs of allergy – redness, itching, and erythema

 NB If 'snap-on' ECG cables are being used with central stud electrodes, connect them up before application to the patient's skin.

ECG monitoring: Trouble shooting

'Flat line' trace

Check if it is asystole – check the patient, although asystole is rarely a straight line. It is usually a mechanical problem. Check:

- ECG monitoring lead selected on monitor, e.g. lead II
- ECG gain (effects size of complexes)
- Electrodes: in date, gel sponge moist, not dry
- ECG cables: connected

 NB Flat line ECG trace: always check the patient first – is it cardiac arrest?

Wandering ECG baseline

This is usually caused by patient movement, particularly respirations. It may help to reposition the electrodes away from the lower ribs.

Electrical interference

This is usually caused by electrical interference from devices by the bedside, e.g. infusion pumps. Remove the source of the interference if possible.

Insecure ECG electrode

A wandering ECG baseline, together with sudden breaks in the signal, suggests an insecure electrode. Ensure:

- Electrodes are positioned correctly
- Skin interface is adequate, i.e. shave excess hair, dry skin if clammy
- ECG cables are not caught and there is no tugging on the electrodes

Small ECG complexes

Pathological causes of small ECG complexes include pericardial effusion, obesity, and hypothyroidism. It may be due to a technical problem:

- Check ECG gain is correctly set
- Select alternative ECG monitoring lead, e.g. lead I
- Try repositioning the electrodes

Unreliable heart rate display on monitor

Ensure there is an adequate ECG trace to avoid:

- Small ECG complexes: false-low heart rate may be displayed
- Large T waves, muscle movement, and interference may be mistaken for QRS complexes and false-high heart rate may be displayed

 Common misinterpretations and pitfalls

The heart rate displayed on the ECG monitor can sometimes be grossly inaccurate: always check the patient.

10 Recording a 12 lead ECG

Introduction

- An electrocardiograph is a machine that records the waveforms generated by the heart's electrical activity
- An electrocardiogram (ECG) is a record or display of a person's heartbeat produced by an electrocardiograph
- Care should be taken to ensure accuracy and standardisation as poor technique can lead to misinterpretation of the ECG, mistaken diagnosis, wasted investigations, and mismanagement of the patient

Indications

- Chest pain
- Myocardial infarction
- Sometimes prior to a general anaesthetic
- Cardiac arrhythmias
- History of collapse/syncope

Procedure

- Identify the patient
- Explain the procedure to the patient
- Assemble the equipment, ensuring that the ECG cables are not twisted as this can cause interference
- Ensure the environment is warm and the patient is relaxed as far as possible. This will help produce a clear, stable trace without interference
- Ensure the patient is lying down in a comfortable position, ideally resting against a pillow at an angle of 45° with the head well supported (an identical patient position should be adopted as with previous 12 lead ECGs: this will help ensure standardisation). The inner aspects of the wrists should be close to, but not touching, the patient's waist

Medical Student Survival Skills: Procedural Skills, First Edition. Philip Jevon and Ruchi Joshi.
© 2020 John Wiley & Sons Ltd. Published 2020 by John Wiley & Sons Ltd.
Companion website: www.wiley.com/go/jevon/medicalstudent

- Prepare the skin if necessary. If wet gel electrodes are used, shaving and abrading the skin is not required. If solid gel electrodes are used, clean/degrease and debrade the skin and shave if necessary
- Apply the electrodes and the limb leads:
  - Red to the inner right wrist
  - Yellow to the inner left wrist
  - Black to the inner right leg, just above the ankle
  - Green to the inner left leg, just above the ankle
- Apply the electrodes to the chest and attach the chest leads:
  - V1 (white/red lead): 4th intercostal space, just to the right of the sternum
  - V2 (white/yellow lead): 4th intercostal space, just to the left of the sternum
  - V3 (white/green lead): midway between V2 and V4
  - V4 (white/brown lead): 5th intercostal space, mid-clavicular line
  - V5 (white/black lead): on anterior axillary line, on the same horizontal line as V4
  - V6 (white/violet lead): mid-axillary line, on the same horizontal line as V4
- Check the calibration signal on the ECG machine to ensure standardisation
- Ask the patient to lie still and breathe normally
- Print out the ECG following the manufacturer's recommendations
- Once an adequate 12 lead ECG has been recorded, disconnect the patient from the ECG machine and clear equipment away and clean as necessary following the manufacturer's recommendations. Sometimes electrodes are left on the patient if serial recordings are going to be required
- Ensure the ECG is correctly labelled. Report and store the ECG in the correct patient's notes following local procedures

 Common misinterpretations and pitfalls

Incorrect connection of the limb leads can lead to misinterpretation of the ECG.

Locating the intercostal spaces for the chest leads

Use the angle of Louis as a reference point for locating the 2nd intercostal space. The procedure is:

- Palpate the angle of Louis (sternal angle) – it is at the junction between the manubrium and the body of the sternum

- Slide the fingers towards the right side of the patient's chest and locate the 2nd rib, which is attached to the angle of Louis
- Slide the fingers down towards the patient's feet and locate the 2nd intercostal space
- Slide the fingers further down to locate the 3rd and 4th ribs and the corresponding four intercostal spaces

 Common misinterpretations and pitfalls

Using the right clavicle as a reference point to palpate the 1st intercostal space can lead to mistaking the space between the clavicle and the 1st rib as the 1st intercostal space.

Alternative chest lead placements

Alternative chest lead placements are sometimes indicated.

- *Right-sided*: used in inferior or posterior myocardial infarction, to ascertain whether there is right ventricular involvement (these patients may require careful management for hypotension and pain relief) and dextrocardia. The chest leads are labelled V3R–V6R and are in effect reflections of the left-sided chest leads V3–V6
- *Posterior*: particularly if there are reciprocal changes in V1–V2, suggesting posterior myocardial infarction. Chest leads are applied to the patient's back below the left scapula, corresponding to the same level as the 5th intercostal space, to view the posterior surface of the heart
- *Higher or more lateral on the chest*: used if the clinical history is suggestive of myocardial infarction, but the ECG is inconclusive

Labelling the 12 lead ECG

- Labelling the 12 lead ECG should follow local protocols (often done electronically)
- All relevant information should be included, i.e. patient details (name, unit number, date of birth), date and time of recording, and ECG serial number, together with any relevant information, e.g. if the patient was free from pain or complaining of chest pain during the recording or after reperfusion therapy
- The leads should be correctly labelled and deviations to the standard recording of a 12 lead ECG should be noted, e.g. right-sided chest leads, paper speed of 50 mm s^{-1}, or different patient position

Standardisation

- To help comparison of serial 12 lead ECGs, they should be recorded with the patient in the same position. If this is not possible (e.g. if the patient has orthopnoea), a note to this effect should be made because the electrical axis of the heart (main direction of current flow) can be altered which makes reviewing and comparing serial ECGs difficult
- Standard calibration is 10 mm to 1 mV vertical deflection on the ECG
- Standard paper speed is 25 mm s^{-1}.

NB Any deviations to the standard procedure for the recording of a 12 lead ECG should be highlighted on the ECG. This will help to avoid possible misinterpretation and misdiagnosis.

What the standard 12 lead ECG records

- The heart generates electrical forces, which travel in multiple directions simultaneously. If the flow of current is recorded in several planes, a comprehensive view of this electrical activity can be obtained
- The standard 12 lead ECG records the electrical activity of the heart from 12 different viewpoints or leads ('leads' are viewpoints of the heart's electrical activity, they do not refer to the cables or wires that connect the patient to the monitor or ECG machine) by attaching 10 leads to the patient's limbs and chest

OSCE Key Learning Points

Recording a 12 lead ECG

✔ Ensure the patient is at 45° (ideally)

✔ Ensure limb ECG lead cables are not mixed up

✔ Carefully locate correct anatomical positions for chest ECG lead cables

✔ Check the calibration of the ECG

✔ Request patient's previous ECGs for comparison

Basic respiratory function tests

11

Introduction

- Spirometry tests allow assessment and diagnosis of common respiratory conditions
- There are two key values that spirometry measures (Figure 11.1):
  - Forced vital capacity (FVC) – this is the total lung volume from maximal inspiration to maximal expiration
  - Forced expiratory volume in 1 second (FEV_1) – the volume forcibly expelled in 1 second
- Values are often expressed as a percentage of the predicted values. Predicted values can be calculated from the patient's sex, age, height, and ethnicity
- Respiratory disease can be obstructive or restrictive in nature. Spirometry is used to help identify the type of disease present (Figure 11.2)

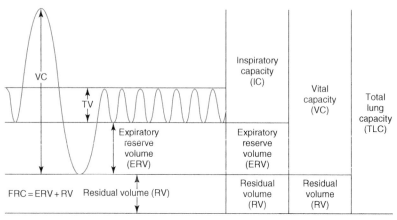

Figure 11.1 Lung volumes. TV (Tidal Volume); FRC (Functional Residual Capacity).

Medical Student Survival Skills: Procedural Skills, First Edition. Philip Jevon and Ruchi Joshi.
© 2020 John Wiley & Sons Ltd. Published 2020 by John Wiley & Sons Ltd.
Companion website: www.wiley.com/go/jevon/medicalstudent

FEV$_1$/FVC ratio

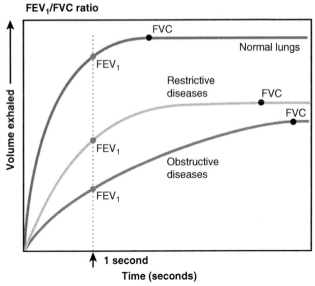

Figure 11.2 Volume–time graph.

Obstructive disease

- FEV$_1$/FVC ratio is reduced to <80%
- FEV$_1$ is reduced
- FVC is reduced or normal

Causes
- Chronic obstructive pulmonary disease (COPD) – normally little reversibility
- Asthma – reversibility seen
- Cystic fibrosis
- Localised airflow obstruction, e.g. with foreign body or tumour

Restrictive disease

- FEV$_1$/FVC ratio is >80%
- FEV$_1$ is reduced
- FVC is reduced

Causes
- Fibrotic lung disease
- Chest wall deformities

- Neuromuscular disease, e.g. motor neurone disease
- Pleural effusion

 NB Mixed defects that comprise an element of both restrictive and obstructive are sometimes present.

Indications

- Diagnosis and monitoring of many common respiratory conditions

Cautions

The results could be affected by many variables such as:
- Acute illnesses, e.g. active infection
- Dementia – inadequate results
- Stress incontinence
- Oral or facial problems affected by mouth piece

Contraindications

- Recent myocardial infarction
- Recent stroke
- Recent surgery – especially eye, thoracic, or abdominal
- Recent pneumothorax
- Haemoptysis

 NB It is advisable for the patient not to smoke or consume alcohol around the time of testing.

Equipment

- Nose clip
- Spirometry machine – multiple different ones are available
- Mouth piece

Procedure

It is unlikely you will have to perform this test yourself but it is always worth understanding what it entails. This will help you understand the results yourself and allow you to explain the test to patients.

NB This test is highly dependent on patient motivation to obtain meaningful results. Ensure the patient has a good seal around the mouth piece and that there are no leaks.

- Sit the patient comfortably. Ensure the chair is at a suitable height for the mouth piece
- Apply the nose clip to occlude the nostrils
- Ask the patient to inspire as much as possible
- The patient is then asked to blow into the mouth piece as fast as possible
- The patient must continue to blow out for as long as possible
- Repeat the process until three similar values are achieved
- Keep the patient sat for some time after as this test can make people feel light headed
- To assess reversibility of disease patients are sometimes given a beta-agonist and retested

OSCE Key Learning Points

✔ This is simple test that allows excellent analysis of the type and severity of respiratory disease

⚠ Common misinterpretations and pitfalls

Spirometry does not diagnose the cause of respiratory disease, just the type, and further investigations may be required.

12 Urine multi-dipstick test

Introduction

- Different types of dipstick can be used to identify and quantify the presence of abnormal components of urine
- If there is an infection, the urine sample can be sent away for further analysis to identify the organisms present and their sensitivities/resistance to antimicrobials; this is called a microscopy, sensitivity, and culture (MC&S) test

Components of a urine dipstick

- Visual inspection
  - Colour
  - Clarity
- pH
- Protein
- Glucose
- Nitrites
- Ketones
- Blood
- Specific gravity (SG)

Colour of urine

- Common causes of discoloured urine include dehydration, medication, and bile pigments

Clarity of urine

- The most common causes of turbid urine are pyuria (pus) or contamination with vaginal epithelial cells or mucous

Medical Student Survival Skills: Procedural Skills, First Edition. Philip Jevon and Ruchi Joshi.
© 2020 John Wiley & Sons Ltd. Published 2020 by John Wiley & Sons Ltd.
Companion website: www.wiley.com/go/jevon/medicalstudent

pH

- Normal range: 4.5–8
- Acidic fruits, uric acid calculi, and metabolic activity can make urine more acidic

Protein

- Normal range: healthy adults excrete approximately 80–150 mg protein in 24 hours
- Proteinuria may indicate interstitial renal disease, renovascular disease, or multiple myeloma

Glucose

- Likely to be raised in undiagnosed/poorly controlled diabetic patients

Nitrites

- May be positive in a bacterial urinary tract infection (UTI)
  - Gram-negative and some Gram-positive bacteria break down nitrates to nitrites
- False positive – reagent is sensitive to air
- False negative – low volume of bacteria or early infection

Ketones

- Positive in states of starvation, pregnancy, and diabetic ketoacidosis

Blood

- Most common false positive is contamination with menstrual blood; other false positives include exercise and dehydration (causing an increase in concentration of red blood cells)
- Not a very sensitive test; best test is microscopy
- Urine dipstick does not differentiate between haematuria, myoglobinuria, or haemoglobinuria

Specific gravity

- Normal range: < 1.008 is dilute; > 1.020 is concentrated
- Low specific gravity indicates a more dilute sample

NB Urine dipsticks only test for one of three ketones produced by the body; acetoacetic acid is detected but beta-hydroxybutyric acid and acetone are not detected.

Indications

- Any symptoms or signs of urinary tract pathology
- Any signs of infection of unknown source or sepsis, e.g. delirium, especially in elderly patients

Equipment

- Urine specimen pot
- Non-sterile gloves
- Urine dipstick
- Results chart for comparison with dipstick
- Patient's results card
- Clinical waste bin

Procedure for dipstick test

Pre-procedure

- Prepare equipment
- Identify correct patient
- Confirm indication for urine dipstick test
- Explain procedure of mid-stream urine specimen (MSU) collection to the patient
- Wash hands and don non-sterile gloves

Procedure

- Note the colour and clarity of the urine sample
- Open urine sample pot; note any offensive smell
- Place dipstick completely into urine sample
- Remove immediately
- Compare dipstick with corresponding coloured square on dipstick results chart (usually on the side of the dipstick container pot) to derive the results (Figure 12.1)

Post-procedure

- Document the results on a urine dipstick card
- Label the card with the patient's details
- Write the results in the patient's notes
- Inform the clinical team of the results if appropriate
- Discard the urine sample and dipstick in the clinical waste bin/sluice if no further analysis is needed

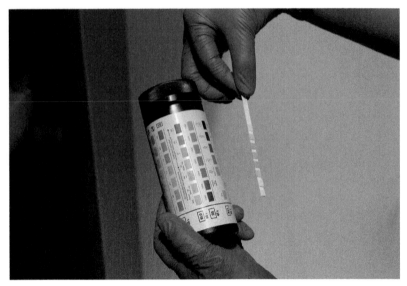

Figure 12.1 Reading the dipstick results.

 NB Do not immediately throw away the sample; if the result is abnormal, you may wish to repeat the dip, send it away for MC&S, and/or perform a pregnancy test on the same sample.

OSCE Key Learning Points

✔ Complete immersion of dipstick
✔ Immediate removal from sample
✔ Correct interpretation

⚠ Common misinterpretations and pitfalls

- Positive urine dipstick or MC&S results do not require treatment with antibiotics unless the patient is symptomatic
- Bacteria from the skin can contaminate the sample if the MSU is incorrectly taken, providing a false-positive result

13 Advising patients on how to collect a mid-stream urine specimen

Introduction

- A mid-stream urine specimen (MSU) is a urine sample that is taken during the middle of the urine stream
- An MSU is used to confirm the diagnosis of a urinary tract infection (UTI), sexually transmitted infection, (STI), and infections during pregnancy. Urine in the bladder should be sterile, so should contain no bacteria
- An MSU can also be sent to the laboratory and cultured to identify if bacteria are present and which antibiotics will respond best in treating the infection
- Urine infections usually cause symptoms of pain on passing urine, and increased urgency and frequency to pass urine
- However, symptoms are not always typical, particularly in children and the elderly, and a urine test is needed. Always check the patient's current symptoms

Indications

- To diagnose UTIs and other infections in the genital tract
- To rule out infection as a cause for other symptoms

Contraindications

- There are no contraindications.

Medical Student Survival Skills: Procedural Skills, First Edition. Philip Jevon and Ruchi Joshi.
© 2020 John Wiley & Sons Ltd. Published 2020 by John Wiley & Sons Ltd.
Companion website: www.wiley.com/go/jevon/medicalstudent

Procedure for MSU test

Pre-procedure

- Explaining the procedure to the patient will ensure they will take the sample correctly
- The first part of the urine can be contaminated with bacteria from the genital area, and the last part of the sample can be contaminated from bacteria in the bladder or higher in the urinary system. Explain to the patient a sample is needed from the middle of their bladder
- A mid-stream sample is a good way of collecting a sample that should be free from bacteria

Procedure

- Prior to providing an MSU, label a sterile container with the name, date of birth, and date of collecting the sample
- Wash hands and genitals
- Men: pull back the foreskin
- Women: hold open the labia (entrance to the vagina)
- Open the lid of the sterile bottle/pot provided by the nurse/doctor
- Void some urine into the toilet and then without stopping the flow of urine, catch some urine in a sterile bottle/pot (Figure 13.1)
- Once there is enough urine in the bottle, void the remaining urine into the toilet
- Seal the cap back on the container
- Wash and dry hands
- Return the sample to the doctor's surgery, or to the laboratory, as soon as possible (within 2 hours is best). If that is not possible, put the sample in the fridge until you take it to the doctor or laboratory
- Allow the patient to summarise the above to ensure they have understood

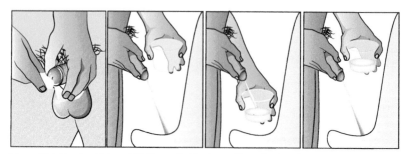

Figure 13.1 How to obtain an MSU in a male. Courtesy of Peter Gardiner/Science Photo Library.

Dos and don'ts

- *Don't* open the sterile bottle until you are ready to take the sample
- *Don't* fill the bottle to the top, a small amount will do. If there is a mark on the bottle it may contain some preservative, in this case you should try and fill the bottle up to this line
- *Don't* touch any part of your genitals with the bottle or unsterile surfaces as this will increase the risk of contamination
- *Do* take the sample to the doctor or laboratory within 24 hours

Results

The result of an MSU takes 2–3 days and will identify whether there is evidence of urinary infection and, if so, which antibiotic will be most suitable for treating the infection.

Complications

- There are no complications.

OSCE Key Learning Points

✔ Explain procedure thoroughly
✔ Summarise procedure
✔ Check patient understanding
✔ Explain results to patient

Introduction

- Swabs are taken from a specific area to innoculate culture medium in the laboratory. This permits identification of the bacteria growing in that area
- Polymerase chain reaction (PCR) can be used to identify viral DNA; this is sometimes done with throat swabs. The procedure for swabbing is the same as the one described below
- Swabs are also taken from the vagina (low and high vaginal swabs) and urethra in males: this is a specialist area beyond the scope of this text, although the principles are the same
- Swabs are taken to sample the bacteria growing in a specific area. It is important that they are not contaminated with bacteria from another area, or another person
- As the bacteria have to be cultured in the lab, swab results take 3–4 days to come back. Bacteria grown from swabs can be tested for their sensitivity to various antibiotics – this is useful when choosing an antibiotic to treat infection
- When interpreting swab results it is important to differentiate between *colonisation* and *infection*
- The surface of the nose, throat, and skin are normally colonised with bacteria: colonisation is asymptomatic
- Deeper tissues (dermis, soft tissue, blood, bone) are normally sterile
- Infection occurs when pathogens invade into the sterile tissues, and cause an inflammatory reaction
- Infection is normally caused by a single species, whereas colonised areas are always colonised with multiple species
- Swabs do not always help to identify the infecting pathogen
- It is common for the normal flora to persist in the area overlying an infected area: in these cases the swab results will fail to identify a pathogen (they may be reported as showing 'mixed growth')

Medical Student Survival Skills: Procedural Skills, First Edition. Philip Jevon and Ruchi Joshi.
© 2020 John Wiley & Sons Ltd. Published 2020 by John Wiley & Sons Ltd.
Companion website: www.wiley.com/go/jevon/medicalstudent

- In infections, the infecting species sometimes predominates in the swabbed area: in these cases the bacterial species grown from the swab is likely to be the pathogen. Antibiotic treatment can be targeted to the likely pathogen

NB Treat the patient, not the swab! 'Mixed growth' on a swab does not exclude infection – it just means your swab has failed to identify the pathogen.

Indications

- Decolonisation treatment is carried out in hospitals and institutions to limit the number of patients colonised with MRSA. MRSA colonisation is not dangerous; MRSA infection is life-threatening
- Patients are swabbed to detect MRSA colonisation when they come into hospital because:
  - Invasive procedures performed in hospital convey an increased risk of patients becoming infected with their own skin commensal bacteria (i.e. MRSA)
  - Healthcare workers may unintentionally transfer MRSA from one patient to another, spreading the risk
- On admission to hospital, the nose and skin (groin) of all patients are swabbed: this is to screen for patients who are colonised with MRSA on their skin
- Swabs are taken from ulcers, wounds, and broken areas of infected skin to identify pathogens causing deeper infection
- Swabs are taken from the throat to identify pathogens causing deeper infection

NB There is no need to swab ulcers or wounds which are healing: if there are no signs of infection, there is no local pathogen!

Cautions

- Swab results may fail to identify a pathogen: failure to isolate a pathogen does not rule out infection
- Conversely, growth of a single dominant species from a swab is not necessarily indicative of infection: it may just predominate in the commensal flora

Contraindications

- Nose: mid-face fractures, base of skull fracture
- Throat: any airway obstruction, oedema, or stridor. If you are concerned the airway may be threatened – do not swab, get help!

Equipment

- Appropriate sterile swab, with associated container (Figure 14.1)
- Tongue depressor
- Non-sterile gloves
- Pen or stickers to label swabs

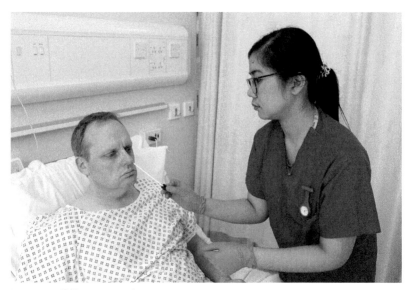

Figure 14.1 Taking a nose swab.

Procedure for insertion

Pre-procedure

- Prepare equipment
- Identify correct patient
- Explain procedure to the patient
- Obtain verbal consent for the procedure
- Wash hands and don non-sterile gloves

Procedure

- *Nose*:
  - Remove the swab from the packet, touching only the plastic end-piece
  - Lightly rub the swab on the inner surface of the nostril
  - Do not insert the swab more than 1 cm into the nostril
  - Place the swab in the container
  - Do not allow the swab to touch anything other than the inner surface of the nostril
- *Throat*:
  - Remove the swab from the packet, touching only the plastic end-piece
  - Sit opposite the patient
  - Warn the patient that swabbing the throat may make them feel slightly uncomfortable: ask them to tap your knee if it is unbearable, and tell them you will stop when they tap your knee
  - Unwrap the swab, and hold the swab in your dominant hand
  - Ask the patient to open their mouth and stick out their tongue
  - Pick up the tongue depressor with your non-dominant hand, and depress the tongue enough so that you can see the tonsils
  - Lightly rub the swab on the tonsil. If only one tonsil is inflamed, rub the swab on the inflamed one
  - Place the swab in the container
  - Do not allow the swab to touch anything other than the tonsil
- *Skin*:
  - Warn the patient that swabbing ulcers or broken skin can be painful – reassure them that you will be gentle, and ask them to tell you if the pain is unbearable and they want you to stop
  - Undress the relevant area. If this is painful, you may want to give some oral analgesia (commonly oral opiates) prior to proceeding
  - Remove the swab from the packet, touching only the plastic end-piece
  - Lightly rub the swab on the relevant area
  - Place the swab in the container
  - Do not allow the swab to touch anything other than the relevant area of skin

Post-procedure

- Thank the patient
- Label the swab's container according to local protocol: some NHS Trusts will have preprinted labels, others will require you to hand-label the container. Whatever system is used, make sure you include:

- Patient identifier (number, name, and date of birth)
- Site the swab was taken from (e.g. ulcer left medial malleolus)
- Date the swab was taken
- Inform the laboratory staff of any antibiotics the patient has been on in the last 72 hours. This is normally done on the form sent with the swab
- Record in the notes that a swab has been taken and sent

OSCE Key Learning Points

✔ Ensure the swab only touches the area of interest
✔ Label the swab accurately and with sufficient information
✔ Do not swab the throat of patients with a compromised airway – you might make it worse
✔ Do not swab the nose of patients with maxillofacial trauma – you could make it much worse

Complications

- If performed correctly in appropriate patients, this is an incredibly safe procedure
- Be careful not to contaminate the swab, e.g. by touching it to an irrelevant area of skin or mucosa

 Common misinterpretations and pitfalls

Growth of a single species of bacteria from a swab does not necessarily indicate infection, nor does failure to isolate a pathogen on a swab indicate that there is no infection: swab results must be interpreted in conjunction with clinical information.

Introduction

Whilst working at the hospital you may have pregnancy as one of your differential diagnoses or you may need to exclude pregnancy to explore alternative diagnoses. A simple and fast way to do this is a human chorionic gonadotrophin (HCG) urine pregnancy test.

HCG is a glycoprotein (hormone) secreted in pregnancy which is made by the developing embryo, and later by the placenta. HCG is essential during pregnancy as it helps maintain hormones such as progesterone, which are needed for the foetus to remain viable. As HCG is excreted in the urine, a urine pregnancy test is the earliest way of detecting a pregnancy.

Principles

HCG is made up of α- and β-subunits. The β-HCG subunit is specific to pregnancy. The HCG pregnancy strips work by using a monoclonal antibody against β-HCG. When the pregnancy strip is immersed in a urine sample, the urine migrates upwards by chromatography to the control area, and then to the test area (if positive) based on the principle of a double antibodies sandwich immunoassay.

HCG pregnancy strips (Figure 15.1) are the most widely available pregnancy tests at most hospitals. Most will have instructions on the back of the packaging.

Recognition of pregnancy

During the early stages there may be some signs/symptoms of pregnancy:
- Missed menstrual period
- Nausea and vomiting

Medical Student Survival Skills: Procedural Skills, First Edition. Philip Jevon and Ruchi Joshi.
© 2020 John Wiley & Sons Ltd. Published 2020 by John Wiley & Sons Ltd.
Companion website: www.wiley.com/go/jevon/medicalstudent

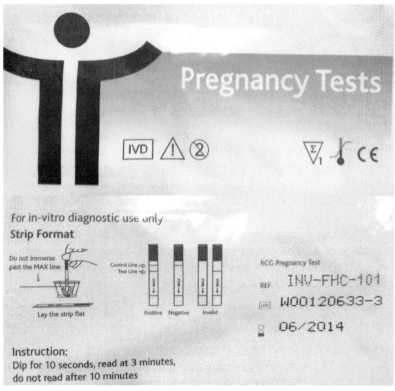

Figure 15.1 The front and back of β-HCG strip packaging made by INVITECH, as used at the Walsall Manor Hospital.

- Tiredness and fatigue
- Increased urination
- Cravings for certain foods

Indications

- To diagnose early pregnancy
- To rule out pregnancy as a cause for other symptoms

Contraindications

- There are no contraindications

Equipment

- Non-sterile gloves and apron
- Urine sample in a container
- Pouch containing pregnancy testing strip
- Watch/timer

Procedure

Pre-procedure

- Prepare equipment needed – check pregnancy test is in-date
- Identify correct patient
- Explain procedure to the patient – collect an early morning sample if possible as it will have the highest concentration of HCG
- Wash hands and put on non-sterile glove

Procedure

- The test strip and urine have to be at room temperature (2–8 °C) for testing
- Remove test strip from the sealed pouch
- Immerse the strip into the urine with the arrow pointing towards the urine. Do not allow the urine level to go over the maximum/marker line (Figure 15.2)
- Take the strip out after 10 seconds and lay flat on a clean, dry surface

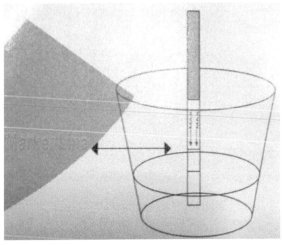

Figure 15.2 The maximum/marker line; urine should not to beyond this line when performing the test.

Post-procedure

- Read the results after 3 minutes
- Ensure the control line is present. Do not read the results after 10 minutes
- Wash hands and dispose of equipment
- Discuss findings with patient
- If an invalid result is found it can be repeated immediately, after 48 hours, or after obtaining an early morning sample

Results

- A colour band/line at the control zone indicates the test has been performed properly
- Negative result: only one colour band appears in the control zone. No apparent band in the test zone means no pregnancy has been detected (Figure 15.3)
- Positive result: two distinct colour bands appear in both the control and test zones (Figure 15.3)
- Invalid: no visible band is seen on the strip or there is an absence of a control band seen regardless of whether there is a test band (Figure 15.3)

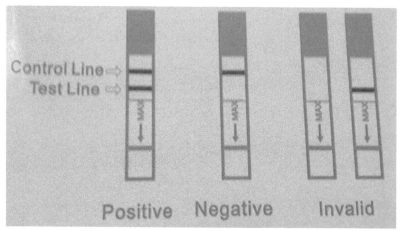

Figure 15.3 The control and test lines showing positive, negative, and invalid results seen on a pregnancy testing strip.

OSCE Key Learning Points

✔ Obtain consent

✔ Insertion of strip in urine sample for 10 seconds

✔ Read results after 3 minutes

✔ Interpret positive, negative, and invalid results

✔ Explain results to patient

Complications

- Unwanted pregnancy
- Ectopic pregnancy – a normal pregnancy cannot be distinguished from an ectopic pregnancy based on HCG levels alone
- False-negative or -positive result – if the sample is too dilute (low specific gravity) it may not contain a representative level of HCG. If the pregnancy is in the very early stages and the HCG is below 25 mIU ml^{-1} a negative result will be shown. If the HCG is very high, it may also present a negative result because of the hook effect
- The HCG test should not be used as a diagnostic tool – HCG levels can be raised in other conditions which must also be ruled out

16 Administering oxygen

Introduction

- Oxygen therapy is the administration of oxygen, in concentrations greater than those in room air to treat hypoxia. These supplementary oxygen concentrations can vary from 24% (nasal cannula) to 95% (non-rebreathe oxygen mask)
- It is important to select the correct oxygen delivery device for the patient, i.e. how much supplementary oxygen needs to be administered and what the patient can actually tolerate
- Oxygen is a colourless, odourless gas that forms about 21% of the earth's atmosphere and is essential for plant and human life
- Tissue oxygenation is dependent upon inspired oxygen, the concentration of haemoglobin, and its ability to saturate with oxygen, as well as the circulation of blood

Indications

Indications for oxygen therapy include:
- Respiratory compromise
- Anaphylaxis
- Shock
- During anaesthesia
- Post surgery

 NB Oxygen therapy should ideally be guided by pulse oximetry.

Medical Student Survival Skills: Procedural Skills, First Edition. Philip Jevon and Ruchi Joshi.
© 2020 John Wiley & Sons Ltd. Published 2020 by John Wiley & Sons Ltd.
Companion website: www.wiley.com/go/jevon/medicalstudent

Components of oxygen therapy

- Oxygen supply: e.g. piped oxygen behind the bed, oxygen cylinder
- Flowmeter: to determine oxygen flow rate in litres/minute
- Oxygen tubing
- Oxygen delivery mechanism: e.g. nasal cannula, non-rebreathe oxygen mask
- Humidifier: to warm and moisten the oxygen prior to administration

Oxygen therapy devices

The oxygen delivery method selected depends on:

- Age of the patient
- Oxygen requirements/therapeutic goals
- Patient tolerance to selected interface
- Humidification requirements

Nasal cannula

A nasal cannula consists of two short prongs which are placed into the patient's nostrils. It is generally well tolerated (less claustrophobic) and does not interfere with eating, drinking, and talking. The nasal cannula is usually only used in patients requiring low percentage concentrations of oxygen, typically flow rates of 2–4 l min^{-1}, achieving inspired oxygen concentrations of 28–35%. Disadvantages include drying of the external mucosal membranes in the nose and irritation of the nostrils.

Fixed oxygen delivery masks (Venturi masks)

Venturi masks enable the delivery of specific oxygen concentrations using a colour-coded Venturi adaptor. These adaptors are colour coded depending on the percentage of oxygen delivered together with the different oxygen flow rates required.

Non-rebreathing oxygen mask

The non-rebreathing oxygen mask (sometimes called a Hudson mask) (Figure 16.1) enables the delivery of high concentrations of oxygen and is recommended for use in acutely ill patients. To ensure the mask is functioning correctly and is effectively used, it is important to follow the manufacturer's recommendations for simple basic checks prior to use. The non-rebreathing mask with an oxygen reservoir bag can be used to deliver high concentrations of oxygen to a spontaneously breathing patient.

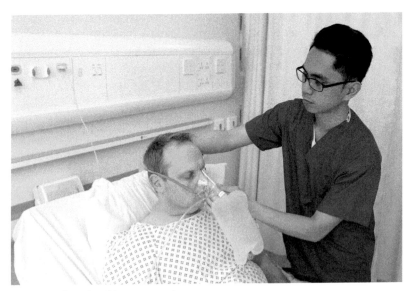

Figure 16.1 Non-rebreathing oxygen mask.

A one-way valve diverts the oxygen flow into the reservoir bag during expiration; the contents of the reservoir bag together with the high-flow oxygen results in minimal entrainment of air and an inspired oxygen concentration of approximately 90%. The valve also prevents the patient's exhaled gases from entering the reservoir bag. The use of the oxygen reservoir bag helps to increase the inspired oxygen concentration by preventing oxygen loss during inspiration.

It is important to ensure that a sufficient oxygen flow rate is used to ensure that the oxygen reservoir bag does not collapse during inspiration. An oxygen flow rate of 12–15 l min^{-1} is recommended. Some non-rebreathing masks have elasticated earloop bands. As these eliminate the need to move the patient's head, they are frequently used in accident and emergency departments for trauma patients.

Procedure

- Ensure the patient is in an upright position to maximise breathing
- Request that pulse oximetry is commenced
- Check the oxygen prescription (see later in this chapter)
- Explain the procedure to the patient
- Attach the oxygen tubing to the oxygen source
- Set the oxygen flow rate to 12–15 l min^{-1}

- Occlude the valve between the mask and the oxygen reservoir bag and check that the reservoir bag is filling up. Remove the finger
- Squeeze the oxygen reservoir bag to check the patency of the valve between the mask and the reservoir bag. If the valve is working correctly it will be possible to empty the reservoir bag (if the reservoir bag does not empty, discard it and select another mask
- Again occlude the valve between the mask and the oxygen reservoir bag, allowing the reservoir bag to fill up
- Place the mask with a filled oxygen reservoir bag on the patient's face, ensuring a tight fit
- Adjust the oxygen flow rate sufficiently to ensure that the reservoir bag deflates by approximately one-third with each breath
- Provide reassurance to the patient
- Closely monitor the patent's vital signs. In particular, assess the patient's response to the oxygen therapy, e.g. respiratory rate, mechanics of breathing, colour, oxygen saturation levels, and level of consciousness. Arterial blood gas analysis will also usually be monitored
- Discontinue/reduce the inspired oxygen concentration as appropriate following advice from a suitably qualified practitioner
- Document the procedure following local protocols

Respiratory rate indicator

Some masks have a respiratory rate indicator to help the healthcare practitioner to monitor the patient's respiratory rate. This indicator can be affected by:

- The patient's respiratory rate
- Orientation of the indicator
- Oxygen flow rate
- Fit of the mask to the patient's face
- Presence of moisture in the indicator tube – this can actually stop the indicator from working

 NB The respiratory rate indicator should only be used as a guide and should not replace close monitoring of the patient's breathing.

Oxygen humidification

Cold, dry air can increase heat and fluid loss. Oxygen has a drying effect on the mucous membranes which can lead to airway damage. In addition, secretions can become thick and difficult to clear. Humidification of long-term oxygen therapy can help prevent these complications. The humidifier should always be positioned below the patient's head.

Prescription of oxygen therapy

Oxygen is a drug and should be prescribed by an appropriately qualified practitioner. This prescription should include:
- Type of oxygen delivery system
- Percentage of oxygen to be delivered (or flow rate)
- Duration of oxygen therapy
- Monitoring that will need to be undertaken

Evidence of harm associated with oxygen therapy

There have been numerous reports of serious incidents relating to inappropriate administration and management of oxygen; of these incidents, poor oxygen management appears to have caused nine patient deaths and may have contributed to a further 35 deaths. Common themes identified from a review of these incidents, local investigations, and other sources are:
- *Prescribing*: failure to prescribe or wrongly prescribed
- *Monitoring*: patients are not monitored, abnormal oxygen saturation levels are not acted upon
- *Administration*: confusion of oxygen with medical compressed air, incorrect flow rates, inadvertent disconnection of supply
- *Equipment*: empty cylinders, faulty and missing equipment

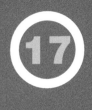

17 Airway management: Insertion of oropharyngeal and nasopharyngeal airways

Introduction

Oropharyngeal and nasopharyngeal airways are useful adjuncts because they can provide an artificial passage to airflow by separating the posterior pharyngeal wall from the tongue.

Oropharyngeal airway

The oropharyngeal airway can be used when there is obstruction of the upper airway due to the displacement of the tongue backwards and when glossopharyngeal and laryngeal reflexes are absent, e.g. during cardiopulmonary resuscitation.

 NB The oropharyngeal airway can only be used if the patient is unconscious.

Cautions

- It should not be used in a patient who is not unconscious as it may induce vomiting and laryngospasm
- It should not be regarded as a definitive airway
- The correct size required should always be estimated
- The correct insertion technique should be adopted to minimise complications

Medical Student Survival Skills: Procedural Skills, First Edition. Philip Jevon and Ruchi Joshi.
© 2020 John Wiley & Sons Ltd. Published 2020 by John Wiley & Sons Ltd.
Companion website: www.wiley.com/go/jevon/medicalstudent

Estimating the correct size

- It is important to estimate the correct size. An oropharyngeal airway that is too big may occlude the airway by displacing the epiglottis, may hinder the use of a face mask, and damage laryngeal structures; while one that is too small may occlude the airway by pushing the tongue back
- An appropriately sized airway is one that holds the tongue in the normal anatomical position and follows its natural curvature
- The curved body of the oropharyngeal airway is designed to fit over the back of the tongue
- The correct size is one that equates to the vertical distance from the angle of the jaw to the incisors; this can be estimated by placing the airway against the face and measuring it from the patient's incisors and the angle of the jaw (Figure 17.1)
- A variety of different sizes are available, although normally sizes 2, 3, and 4 are adequate for small, medium, and large adults, respectively (Figure 17.2)

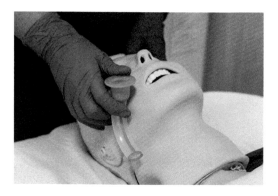

Figure 17.1 Measuring an oropharyngeal airway.

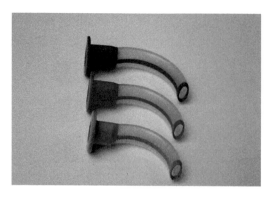

Figure 17.2 Three sizes of oropharyngeal airways.

Procedure for insertion

The correct insertion technique should be used in order to avoid unnecessary trauma to the delicate tissues in the mouth and inadvertently blocking the airway.

- Select an appropriately sized airway
- Lubricate the airway if possible
- Open the patient's mouth and suction if necessary
- Insert the airway into the mouth in the inverted position (Figure 17.3)
- Rotate it through 180° as it passes over the soft palate. The curved part of the airway will help depress the tongue and prevent it from being pushed posteriorly
- Confirm adequate placement of the airway: airway patency should be improved and the flattened reinforced section should be positioned in between the patient's teeth or gums if edentulous
- Following insertion, monitor the patency of the airway and maintain head tilt/chin lift if required
- Periodically reassess the position of the airway as it can easily become dislodged

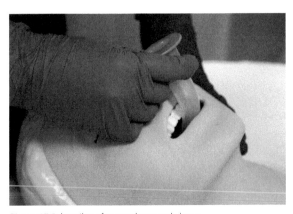

Figure 17.3 Insertion of an oropharyngeal airway.

Nasopharyngeal airway

- The nasopharyngeal airway is made from soft plastic with a flange at one end and a bevelled edge at the other
- It is less likely to induce gagging than an oropharyngeal airway and it can be used in a semiconscious or conscious patient when the airway is at risk of being compromised (e.g. in the post resuscitation period)

- It can be life-saving in a patient with a clenched jaw, trismus, or maxillofacial injuries
- Its use is contraindicated if there is a suspected base of skull fracture as it may penetrate the cranial fossa
- Insertion may damage the mucosal lining of the nasal airway, resulting in bleeding. The correct size should be used and, prior to insertion, a safety pin should be securely inserted into the flange to prevent inhalation of the airway (Figure 17.4)

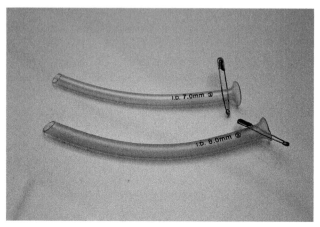

Figure 17.4 Two sizes of nasopharyngeal airways.

Estimating the correct size

- It is important to estimate the correct size. If it is too short it will be ineffective, and if it is too long it may enter the oesophagus causing distension and hypoventilation or may stimulate the laryngeal or glossopharyngeal reflexes causing laryngospasm and vomiting
- The tubes are sized in millimetres according to their internal diameter. Sizes 6–7 are suitable for adults
- Some devices require a safety pin to be inserted through the flange (a precautionary measure to prevent inhalation of the airway)

Procedure for insertion

- Where appropriate explain the procedure to the patient
- Select an appropriately sized airway
- If necessary, insert a safety pin through the flange
- Check the right nostril for patency

- Lubricate the airway
- Insert the airway into the nostril, bevelled end first (Figure 17.5). Pass it vertically along the floor of the nose, using a slight twisting action, into the posterior pharynx (if there is resistance remove the airway and try the left nostril). Once inserted the flange should be at the level of the nostril
- Secure the airway with tape
- Reassess the airway and check for patency and adequacy of ventilation. Continue to maintain correct alignment of the airway and chin lift as necessary and monitor the patency of the airway

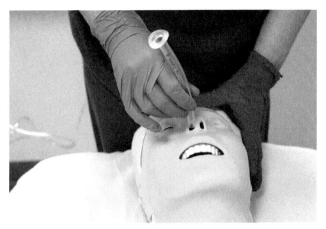

Figure 17.5 Insertion of a nasopharyngeal airway.

 Common misinterpretations and pitfalls

Inserting an oropharyngeal or nasopharyngeal airway does not mean the airway is secure.

Ventilation: Pocket mask and self-inflating bag

18

Introduction

Failure of the circulation for 3–4 minutes (less if the patient is initially hypoxaemic) can lead to irreversible cerebral damage. Restarting the heart following a cardiac arrest may not be possible without adequate reoxygenation. Effective airway management and ventilation during cardiopulmonary resuscitation (CPR) is therefore paramount.

NB The most common cause of failure to ventilate is improper positioning of the head and neck.

Mouth to mouth ventilation

- It is rarely necessary to have to perform mouth to mouth resuscitation, certainly in the hospital environment. At the very least a pocket mask should always be immediately available
- It must be stressed that although mouth to mouth ventilation is effective, it is only possible to deliver oxygen at 16–17% to the patient; a ventilatory device with supplementary oxygen should be used as soon as practically possible

Mouth to mask ventilation (pocket mask)

- The pocket mask is an excellent first response device. It is transparent, thus enabling prompt detection of vomit or blood in the patient's airway
- A one-way valve directs the patient's expired air away from the operator

Medical Student Survival Skills: Procedural Skills, First Edition. Philip Jevon and Ruchi Joshi.
© 2020 John Wiley & Sons Ltd. Published 2020 by John Wiley & Sons Ltd.
Companion website: www.wiley.com/go/jevon/medicalstudent

- Most pocket masks have an oxygen connector for the attachment of supplementary oxygen (15lmin⁻¹), enabling an inspired oxygen concentration of approximately 50% to be achieved
- If there is no oxygen connector, supplementary oxygen can still be added by placing the oxygen tubing underneath one side of the mask and pressing down to achieve a seal

Procedure for mouth to mask ventilation

- Don gloves (if available)
- Kneel behind the patient's head, ensuring the knees are a shoulder-width apart (if alone kneel at the side of the patient, level with their nose and mouth)
- Rest back to sit on the knees and adopt a low kneeling position
- Bend forwards from the hips, leaning down towards the patient's face and resting your elbows on your legs to support your weight
- If available, attach oxygen to the oxygen connector on the mask at a rate of 15lmin⁻¹. If there is no oxygen connector, place the oxygen tubing underneath one side of the mask and press down to achieve a seal
- Apply the mask to the patient's face; press down with the thumbs and lift the chin into the mask by applying pressure behind the angles of the jaw (Figure 18.1)
- Take a breath in and ventilate the patient with sufficient air to cause a visible chest rise. Each ventilation should last 1 second

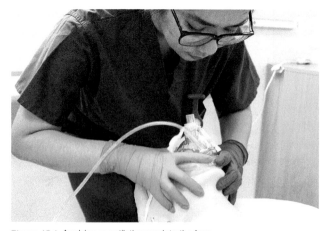

Figure 18.1 Applying a ventilation mask to the face.

- If the patient is on a bed or trolley (its height should already have been adjusted so that the patient is level between the knee and mid-thigh of the nurse performing chest compressions): stand at the side facing the patient, level with their nose and mouth, and bend forwards from the hips to minimise flexion of the spine; the nurse's weight can also be supported by resting their elbows on the bed and leaning their legs against the side of the bed frame. If a colleague is performing chest compressions adopt a position at the top of the bed facing the patient
- Always adopt a comfortable position for ventilation and avoid static postures

Bag–mask ventilation

- The bag–mask (self-inflating bag) device allows the delivery of higher concentrations of oxygen. If an oxygen reservoir bag is attached, with an oxygen flow rate of $15 \, l \, min^{-1}$, an inspired oxygen concentration of approximately 90% can be achieved
- Its use by a single person requires considerable skill. When used with a face mask, it can be difficult to achieve a seal with the mask, maintain an open airway, and squeeze the bag. A two-person technique is therefore recommended, one person to open the airway and ensure a good seal with the mask, while the other squeezes the bag (Figure 18.2)

Procedure for bag–mask ventilation

- Ensure the patient is supine
- Move the bed away from the wall and remove the backrest if applicable. Ensure the brakes of the bed are on. The height of the bed should be adjusted so that the patient is level between the knee and mid-thigh of the nurse performing chest compressions
- Adopt a position at the top of the bed facing the patient, with the feet in a walk/stand position
- Select an appropriately sized mask, i.e. it comfortably covers the mouth and nose, but does not cover the eyes or override the chin
- Ensure an oxygen reservoir bag is attached and connect oxygen at a flow rate of $10 \, l \, min^{-1}$
- First nurse: tilt the head back, apply the mask to the face, pressing down on it with the thumbs. Lift the chin into the mask by applying pressure behind the angles of the jaw. An open airway and an adequate face/mask seal should now be achieved. A pillow under the head and shoulders can help to maintain this position

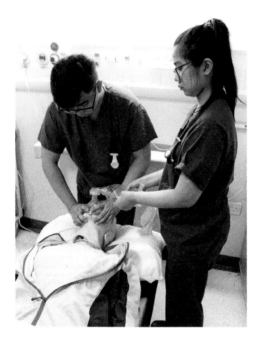

Figure 18.2 Two-person technique for bag–mask ventilation.

- Second nurse (positioned to the side of the bed): squeeze the bag (not the oxygen reservoir bag) sufficiently to cause visible chest rise. Each ventilation should be delivered over 1 second
- Observe for chest rise and fall. If the chest does not rise recheck the patency of the airway; slight readjustment may be all that is required
- Adopt a comfortable position for ventilation and avoid static postures. Supporting your weight by resting your elbows on the bed may help

Minimising gastric inflation

- Excessive tidal volumes or inspiratory flows can generate excessive airway pressures, which can lead to gastric inflation and the subsequent risk of regurgitation and aspiration of gastric contents
- It is therefore recommended to deliver each ventilation over 1 second, with sufficient volume to achieve chest rise, but avoiding rapid and forceful ventilations

Common misinterpretations and pitfalls

If ventilations fail to achieve chest rise:

- Ensure adequate head tilt and chin lift
- Recheck the patient's mouth and remove any obstruction
- Ensure there is a good seal between the mask and the patient's face

OSCE Key Learning Points

Ventilation

✔ Ensure head tilt/chin lift

✔ Ensure airtight seal with mask

✔ Attach oxygen at a flow rate of $15\,l\,min^{-1}$

✔ Check for chest rise following ventilation

19 Defibrillation (manual and automated)

Introduction

Defibrillation describes the method of applying a current to the myocardium to correct an abnormal cardiac rhythm. Being able to recognise and rapidly correct sinister cardiac rhythms is an essential skill that all doctors should be able to perform. However, it goes without saying that should you find yourself considering use of the defibrillator then it is essential to seek senior help urgently.

Background information

- There are two types of defibrillation waveforms which are in use in the United Kingdom. Monophasic defibrillators cause a single waveform when discharged, where the current is applied through the chest from one electrode to the other. Biphasic defibrillators cause both a positive and negative deflection (Figure 19.1). The advantage of biphasic waveforms is that a lower energy setting can be used, reducing the risk of damage to the cardiac myocytes
- Most British hospitals use 'hands-free' defibrillator pads. These are simple adhesive electrodes that are applied to the patient's chest. The main advantage is that the cardiac rhythm can be monitored continuously via the pads rather than via an additional three lead electrocardiogram. You may occasionally see defibrillator paddles used in some hospitals, particularly in cardiac care units – the principle of using these devices is exactly the same as hands-free defibrillation, however care must be taken to avoid inadvertently discharging the current
- Some units use automated external defibrillators (AEDs). They are extremely simple to use, with voice instructions that explain exactly what steps are required. Some even provide an auditory prompt (similar to a metronome) which will help with the timing of chest compressions

Medical Student Survival Skills: Procedural Skills, First Edition. Philip Jevon and Ruchi Joshi.
© 2020 John Wiley & Sons Ltd. Published 2020 by John Wiley & Sons Ltd.
Companion website: www.wiley.com/go/jevon/medicalstudent

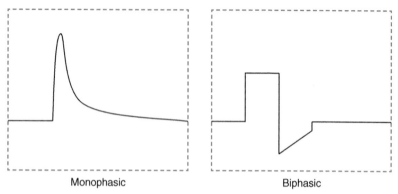

Monophasic   Biphasic

Figure 19.1 Monophasic and biphasic defibrillation waveforms.

Indications

- Ventricular fibrillation (VF) – this is easily identified by its coarse, bizarre waveform
- Pulseless ventricular tachycardia (VT) – this appears as a monomorphic broad complex tachycardia

Cautions

- Torsade de pointes – this appears as a polymorphic VT with a characteristic twisting of the QRS complex around the baseline. It is a recognised complication of long QT syndrome. Patients may initially have a pulse, however it is associated with degenerating into VF. This should be treated initially with intravenous magnesium sulphate, but defibrillation may be required should the patient deteriorate
- Unstable tachycardia (with pulse) – this is defined as a tachycardia with adverse features (shock/syncope/heart failure). *It is essential that if a decision is made to deliver a shock that the waveform is synchronised to the patient's rhythm – otherwise this may lead to pulseless VT/VF.* There is usually a 'sync' button that is present if the defibrillator is able to do this

Contraindications

Defibrillation will not be effective in asystolic patients and should not be attempted.

Equipment

- Hands-free pads
- Defibrillator
- Personal protective equipment

Defibrillation procedure (manual)

Pre-procedure

- Get help (or at least make sure help is coming urgently)
- If there is a cardiac arrest situation, start cardiopulmonary resuscitation (CPR) following the Resuscitation Council (UK) guidelines
- Ensure that there is full resuscitation equipment available
- Intravenous access is a must, but do not let this delay giving the shock

Procedure

- Attach the defibrillation pads: one pad should be placed adjacent to the inferior border of the right clavicle, and the right sternal edge, and the other centred on the 5th intercostal space in the mid-axillary line
- Rhythm check: 'Please stop CPR so that I can assess the rhythm'
- If CPR is in progress ask the team to stop CPR briefly whilst you assess the rhythm. This should only take 2–3 seconds maximum
- Charge the defibrillator: 'A shock is advised. Please continue CPR whilst the machine is charging – I will not shock you'
- If a shockable rhythm is present, inform the team clearly that you intend to deliver a shock. Tell the person doing CPR to continue whilst the machine is charging, and that you will not shock them. Charging typically takes 5–6 seconds.
- Safety check: 'Stand clear of the bed. Oxygen away'
- Tell the team to stand clear, and take the oxygen away from the patient (it is flammable). Check that the trolley is clear at the top, side, and bottom. Finally, check that you are not touching the trolley yourself
- Deliver the shock: 'Shock delivered, resume CPR'
- Finally, press the button to discharge the current. Immediately resume CPR with no delay

Post-procedure

- Follow the Resuscitation Council (UK) guidelines

Defibrillation procedure (automated external defibrillation)

Pre-procedure

- Get help (or at least make sure help is coming urgently)
- If there is a cardiac arrest situation, follow the Resuscitation Council (UK) guidelines
- Ensure that there is full resuscitation equipment available
- Intravenous access is a must, but do not let this delay giving the shock

Procedure

- Turn on the AED, and attach the defibrillation pads: one pad should be placed adjacent to the inferior border of the right clavicle, and the right sternal edge, and the other centred on the 5th intercostal space in the mid-axillary line. There will usually be a diagram on the pads to help you
- Rhythm check: the AED will verbally tell the team to stop CPR briefly whilst it assesses the rhythm
- If a shockable rhythm is present, the machine will verbally confirm the presence of an arrhythmia and inform the team that it intends to deliver a shock. It will charge automatically which typically takes 5–6 seconds. Follow the machine's instructions closely – do not touch the patient when the shock is being delivered!
- Continue CPR for 2 minutes: the machine will then tell the team to continue CPR for another cycle. Some brands use a metronome sound to indicate the speed of chest compression, but make sure that the depth is also adequate. At the end of the 2 minutes, the machine will ask the team to stop CPR for a rhythm check – this will be done automatically

Post-procedure

- Follow the Resuscitation Council (UK) guidelines

OSCE Key Learning Points

- ✔ Take the time to familiarise yourself with the defibrillator in your clinical environment
- ✔ If you are not familiar with the equipment, use the maximum possible energy level
- ✔ Do not stop chest compressions whilst the machine is charging – each second without effective compressions severely compromises the chance of a successful outcome

20 Cardiopulmonary resuscitation

Introduction

- Cardiopulmonary resuscitation (CPR) is an emergency procedure performed during a cardiac arrest in an attempt to re-establish circulation and breathing
- The Resuscitation Council (UK) in-hospital algorithm (Figure 20.1) provides guidance for in-hospital resuscitation
- CPR is performed to keep a patient alive until a reversible cause can be treated and advanced emergency care can be provided
- With most patients displaying adverse signs prior to cardiac arrest, the recognition of acute illness, together with effective treatment and appropriate management following the ABCDE approach to prevent deterioration is paramount

NB In 80% of in-hospital cardiac arrests patients have displayed adverse signs prior to collapse.

Cardiac arrest rhythms

- Ventricular fibrillation
- Pulseless ventricular tachycardia
- Pulseless electrical activity
- Asystole

Cardiac arrest team

- The team usually comprises a senior doctor (e.g. resident medical officer), junior doctors, an anaesthetist, resuscitation officer, and a senior nurse, (e.g. critical care unit nurse)
- One person should be the team leader

Medical Student Survival Skills: Procedural Skills, First Edition. Philip Jevon and Ruchi Joshi.
© 2020 John Wiley & Sons Ltd. Published 2020 by John Wiley & Sons Ltd.
Companion website: www.wiley.com/go/jevon/medicalstudent

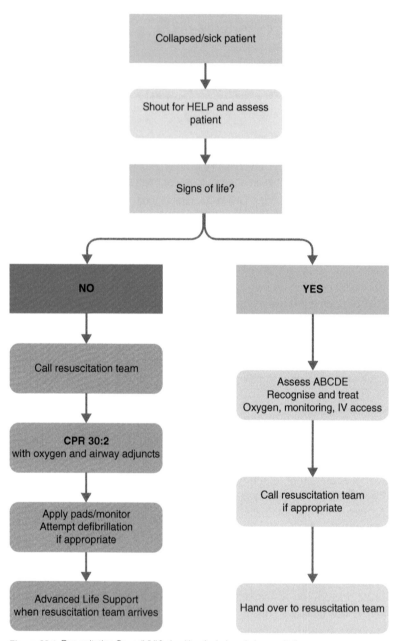

Figure 20.1 Resuscitation Council (UK) algorithm for in-hospital resuscitation.

Reversible causes of cardiac arrest

In every cardiac arrest it is important to exclude eight potentially reversible causes (four 'H's and four 'T's):

- Hypoxia
- Hypoglycaemia
- Hypothermia
- Hyperkalaemia
- Thromboembolism
- Toxins (i.e. poisoning)
- Tension pneumothorax
- Tamponade (cardiac)

Equipment

- Non-sterile gloves
- Other protective equipment may be required – aprons, face masks
- Fully stocked cardiac arrest (or crash) trolley following Resuscitation Council (UK) guidelines

Procedure

In the event of a collapsed or unresponsive patient follow this procedure.

Safety

- Ensure personal safety and check patient surroundings are safe
- Ensure safety of team
- Use of personal protective equipment, e.g. gloves
- Take care with sharps, etc. – sharps box should be on the crash trolley
- Use safe moving and handling techniques

Check for response

- Shake and shout: check response (Figure 20.2)
- If no response: call for help, active emergency button, etc. (Figure 20.3)

Check for signs of life

- Take no more than 10 seconds to determine if a patient is in cardiac arrest
- Look for signs of life – purposeful movement, coughing, normal breathing (Figure 20.4)

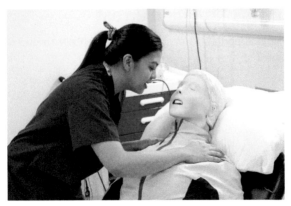

Figure 20.2 Check patient's response.

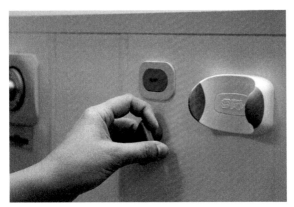

Figure 20.3 Activate the emergency button.

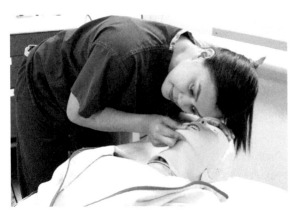

Figure 20.4 Check for signs of life and signs of normal breathing.

- Open the airway using a head tilt and chin lift and assess for breathing:
  - Look for movement of the chest and abdomen
  - Listen at the mouth and nose for breath sounds
  - Feel at the mouth and nose for airflow on your cheek

 Common misinterpretations and pitfalls

Agonal breathing is a sign of early cardiac arrest. Agonal breathing is very slow and laboured breathing and/or occasional gasps. Do not mistake agonal breathing for normal breathing.

- If trained to do so, while checking for signs of normal breathing, palpate the carotid pulse at the same time

Start CPR

- If there are no signs of life and no signs of normal breathing, start CPR immediately, with chest compressions first
- Ask a colleague to call the cardiac arrest team (usually by dialling 2222)
- Send for cardiac arrest trolley and defibrillator

Chest compressions

- CPR should be commenced immediately after confirming cardiac arrest
- CPR is performed at ratio of 30 chest compressions to two ventilations. In practice, in-hospital chest compressions will be performed continuously until colleagues are ready to ventilate using a bag–valve–mask device. Mouth to mouth is not usually undertaken in the hospital environment
- When performing chest compressions:
  - Ensure the patient is flat on a hard surface, e.g. a bed, which is at a suitable height for the person performing the chest compressions (patient should be roughly at the level of the person's knee to mid-thigh (Figure 20.5)
  - Place the one hand (usually the dominant hand) in the middle of the lower half of the sternum; place your other hand on top of your first hand and interlock your fingers (Figure 20.6)
  - Compress the chest 5–6 cm at a rate of 100–120 compressions per minute
- Start the next compression once the chest has completely recoiled
- Minimise any interruptions to chest compressions

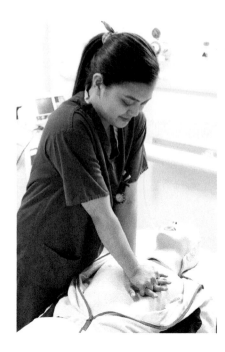

Figure 20.5 Performing chest compressions.

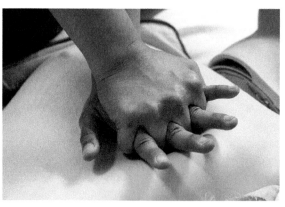

Figure 20.6 Position of hands in performing chest compressions.

 NB Performing chest compressions can be very tiring. If there are a sufficient number of rescuers, ensure changing of the person doing chest compressions every 2 minutes with minimal interruptions to compressions.

Defibrillation

- As soon as the defibrillator arrives, switch it on and follow the instructions
- Attach defibrillation pads to the patient's bare chest as soon as possible
- Defibrillate if indicated/advised (Figure 20.7)

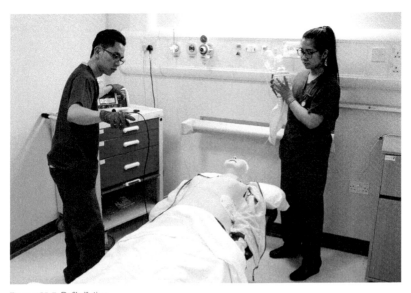

Figure 20.7 Defibrillation.

 NB If the patient needs defibrillating, for every minute defibrillation is delayed the chance of the patient being discharged alive from hospital plummets by about 10%.

Ventilations

- Perform airway opening manoeuvres – head tilt and chin lift or a jaw thrust
- Maintain an open airway using simple adjuncts, e.g.
  - Oropharyngeal/Guedel airway
  - Supraglottic airway, e.g. laryngeal mask airway- LMA

 NB If there is a risk of cervical spine injury, manual in-line stabilisation of the head and neck should be performed throughout resuscitation.

- Use available equipment for ventilation:
  - Pocket mask (Figure 20.8)
  - Bag–valve–mask device (Figure 20.9)
- Ventilations should have an inspiratory time of 1 second, and provide sufficient inspiratory volume to produce a visible rise in the patient's chest

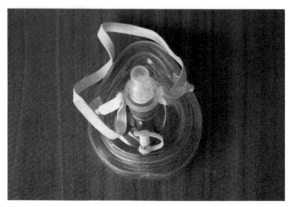

Figure 20.8 Pocket mask.

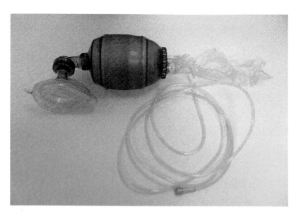

Figure 20.9 Bag–valve–mask device.

 NB Endotracheal intubation should only be performed by trained and competent healthcare professionals. Once an endotracheal airway has been placed, chest compressions are performed continuously with simultaneous ventilations at 10 breaths min^{-1}.

Advanced life support

- Continue CPR until the arrival of the resuscitation team. If there is sufficient staff and equipment, establish intravenous access and prepare drugs likely to be used in resuscitation (e.g. adrenaline)
- Identify and treat reversible causes of cardiac arrest)
- Every 2 minutes, the electrocardiogram should be reassessed

OSCE Key Learning Points

Priorities in an in-hospital cardiac arrest

✔ Recognise cardiac arrest immediately

✔ Call 2222 for cardiac arrest team

✔ Start chest compressions

✔ Defibrillate (if indicated) as soon as possible

21 Establishing peripheral intravenous access

Introduction

- A peripheral IV cannula is a short, plastic tube introduced into a vein over a needle
- It is the most commonly used form of vascular access in medicine, allowing the administration of treatments directly to the bloodstream where treatments can exert their quickest and maximal effects

Indications

Common indications for securing IV access include:
- Administration of fluids
- Administration of medications, e.g. antibiotics
- Blood transfusion
- Contrast media for imaging
- Prophylactically due to the potential for deterioration, before a procedure, or if the patient is unlikely to be able to safely swallow

Contraindications

- *Relative contraindications*:
  - Bleeding tendency
- *Absolute contraindications*:
  - Inflammation, infection, or skin breakdown at site of cannulation
  - Arteriovenous fistula in arm of proposed site
  - Previous mastectomy with axillary node clearance on same side of intended upper limb cannulation
  - Lower limbs of diabetic patients

Medical Student Survival Skills: Procedural Skills, First Edition. Philip Jevon and Ruchi Joshi.
© 2020 John Wiley & Sons Ltd. Published 2020 by John Wiley & Sons Ltd.
Companion website: www.wiley.com/go/jevon/medicalstudent

This is not a rigid guide. In extremis, IV access is *always* preferred regardless of location.

The IV cannula

- A cannula is composed of several parts, notably the needle, catheter, wings, injection port, and cap. Most cannulas also have a flashback chamber to show that the device has entered a vein
- It is important to select the correct size cannula for the clinical indication (Table 21.1). The flow rate of the cannula is proportional to the length and the radius of the inner tube (to the fourth power). Thus, a small change in the internal radius can have a profound increase in flow rate, e.g. doubling of the internal radius results in a 16× increase in flow rate
- Certain drugs can irritate veins, and so must be infused via a cannula placed into a large vein or via a central venous catheter, e.g. 50% glucose

Table 21.1 Selecting the Correct Size Cannula for the Clinical Indication

Colour	Size (gauge)	Maximal flow rate	Typical uses
Blue	22	36 ml min^{-1}	Children, small fragile vein, elderly patients
Pink	20	61 ml min^{-1}	IV maintenance fluids, drugs
Green	18	90 ml min^{-1}	Blood transfusion
White	17	140 ml min^{-1}	Rapid infusions of fluids, drugs, and blood products. Commonly used in theatres during long operations
Grey	16	200 ml min^{-1}	
Brown/orange	14	300 ml min^{-1}	Emergency transfusion of blood/fluids and drugs

Choosing the site of cannulation

Factors to consider when placing a cannula:
- Patient comfort
- Convenience of access
- Size of cannula required
- Size, mobility, and fragility of veins
- Clinical indication
- Length of time cannula to remain in situ

Sites for cannulation

 NB Where possible use the non-dominant side.

- Dorsum of hand – comfortable, easily accessed and inspected, lowest risk of phlebitis
- Forearm – easily accessed and inspected, large veins
- Antecubital fossa – large veins, but less easy to access and inspect, less comfortable, likely to obstruct flow when elbow is flexed

Theoretically, a cannula may be placed into any vein that will accept one, but practical aspects tend to result in the above sites being chosen.

Equipment list

- Tourniquet
- Skin preparation (usually a chlorhexidine wipe or applicator)
- Appropriate cannula
- IV dressing
- Sharps bin
- 10 ml syringe
- 10 ml 0.9% sodium chloride

Procedure for IV cannulation

As with any clinical skill, it is important to fully explain the procedure to the patient and gain consent. Set up a sterile field, and wear an apron and non-sterile gloves.

- Position the patient comfortably so that the vein or area of interest is exposed. Ensure lighting is adequate
- Apply a tourniquet proximally above the area of interest
- Look and feel for appropriate veins. A suitable vein is full and bouncy when palpated. It may not be visible. Look for sites where veins branch into two – just proximal to this is usually an ideal site for cannulation
- Clean the area and allow to dry. Do not palpate the skin following this
- Remove the cannula cap and set aside
- With your non-dominant hand, firmly immobilise the vein and pull the skin taut below the site of insertion. Grasp the cannula in your dominant hand
- Warn the patient that they will experience a sharp sting as you begin to pass the cannula
- Introduce the cannula to the skin at an angle of no more than 30°. Advance in the direction of the vein. There is a characteristic 'feel' when entering the lumen. This will come with experience

- When flashback in seen in the cannula chamber (primary flashback), advance the cannula a few more millimetres to ensure it is in the lumen of the vein. Do not advance too far, as the cannula will puncture the posterior wall of the vein
- Withdraw the needle from the cannula and observe secondary flashback along the plastic sheath. If no flashback is seen, adjust the position of the cannula
- Advance the cannula into the vein whilst holding the needle
- Remove the tourniquet
- Occlude the vein proximally with a finger and place gauze at the open end of the cannula to catch any blood drops when the needle is removed
- Remove the needle and dispose of it into the sharps bin
- Place the cannula cap onto the cannula
- Secure the cannula with the IV dressing
- Clearly date the cannula with the provided label on the dressing
- Flush the cannula with 10 ml of 0.9% sodium chloride. Observe for any swelling or pain which indicates that the cannula is not properly placed and will need to be removed
- Document the procedure onto the relevant paperwork, usually a visual infusion phlebitis (VIP) chart kept at the point of care

Complications

- Pain – topical or local anaesthetic can be used to facilitate the procedure
- Haematoma formation – a collection of blood may form as the vein is punctured, or soon after. The cannula must be removed and pressure applied to the area for 3–5 minutes
- Inability to advance due to valves – palpation can sometimes detect valves within veins, indicating that they should be avoided. Valves can sometimes be opened by flushing the cannula with normal saline as they are advanced
- Arterial cannulation – occurs most frequently at the antecubital fossa or when cannulating the cephalic vein. It may be disastrous if left unrecognised or if drugs are administered. Signs that an artery has been cannulated include bright red, high-pressure flashback and a pulsing cannula. If in doubt, remove the cannula and apply pressure for at least 5 minutes
- Extravasation – fluids leak into the subcutaneous tissues surrounding the vein, usually because the cannula has become dislodged. The cannula will need to be removed and resited

- Phlebitis – inflammation of the vein. Occurs in around 1/3000 cannulations. May be associated with thrombus formation in a vein. In either case, the cannula must be removed and resited, avoiding the vein in question. Advice should be sought for treatment of the condition

Useful tips

- Ensure the area is well lit, regardless of time of day!
- Spend time selecting a good vein/site
- When cannulating the hand or upper limb, ask the patient to open/close a fist and to hang the arm below the level of the heart to encourage filling
- Tapping the vein gently will encourage vasodilation
- Submerging the hand in warm water or using a tight-fitting glove can encourage vasodilation if you are really struggling
- In the oedematous patient, squeezing oedema away will buy enough time to visualise a vein to cannulate. Beware that oedema will quickly return, so have equipment to hand

---

OSCE Key Learning Points

✔ Warn patient about pain
✔ Ensure infection control measures
✔ Insert cannula in non-dominant hand
✔ Take care with sharps

22 Use of infusion devices

Introduction

- An infusion device is a piece of equipment that allows delivery of fluid or medications at a set rate
- Infusion devices can be used to infuse fluids or medications intravenously, subcutaneously, or intrathecally
- There are various brands and models but there are two main types
- Volumetric devices deliver fluids or medicines from a bag at a set rate (Figure 22.1)

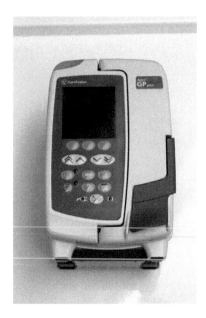

Figure 22.1 Volumetric device.

Medical Student Survival Skills: Procedural Skills, First Edition. Philip Jevon and Ruchi Joshi.
© 2020 John Wiley & Sons Ltd. Published 2020 by John Wiley & Sons Ltd.
Companion website: www.wiley.com/go/jevon/medicalstudent

- Syringe pump deliver medications from a syringe at a set rate (Figure 22.2)

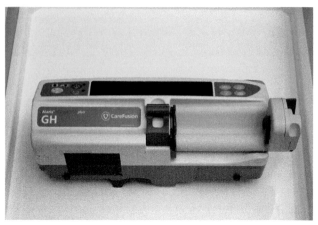

Figure 22.2 Syringe pump.

- Syringe driver – this a portable device that infuses medication, usually subcutaneously or intravenously. They are good in patients requiring continuous medication outside the hospital setting, e.g. palliative analgaesia or continuous insulin administration
- Intravenous and subcutaneous fluids and medications are frequently prescribed to hospital in-patients. Prescription is generally documented on an IV Infusion regime sheet. Included in the prescription is:
  - The type of fluid
  - Additional drug and dose to be added to the fluid if applicable
  - Rate of flow
  - Prescriber's signature
  - The infusion device is used to deliver the intravenous or subcutaneous prescription at a set rate

Indications

Infusion devices may be used in any medical condition where fluid or medication needs to be administered at a set rate. For example:

- Administration of IV fluids in a patient who is dehydrated or nil by mouth
- Administration of IV or subcutaneous medications at a set rate. Most commonly:
  - IV insulin in a patient with diabetic ketoacidosis or hyperglycaemia
  - Subcutaneous morphine or antiemetic in palliative or postoperative patients

Cautions

- Ensure you are trained in use of the particular infusion device you intend to use
- Administer IV fluids with caution in patients with heart disease and the elderly

Contraindications

- There are no absolute contraindications to the use of IV or subcutaneous fluids

Equipment

- Infusion device required
- Prescription of fluid/medication to be infused
- Giving set/infusion line compatible for device

Procedure for infusion

Setting up the infusion

- Ensure you have the correct prescription for the correct patient
- Calculate the rate that this is to be given at. Get another colleague to double check your calculation.
- Wash your hands and don non-sterile gloves
- Connect the giving set/administration line to the fluid/medication.
- Attach the medication/fluid to the IV infusion device.
- Prime the line (run some of the solution through the administration line to the end until it is dripping out)
- Explain procedure to the patient and gain consent
- Check the patient's identification and allergy details against the prescription chart and medication (the safety triangle)
- Attach the administration line to the patient (either to an IV cannula or via a subcutaneous cannula).
- Enter the rate of infusion into the machine. Always do this with the assistance of another colleague to double check.

 NB Only use administration sets compatible with the model you are using.

Monitoring

- Monitor the infusion 10 minutes after starting
- Check the infusion site for signs of extravasation
- Check that the volume in the bag/syringe has reduced
- Check the patient is comfortable

23 Making up drugs for parenteral administration

Introduction

- Drugs are administered through a parenteral route for rapid or direct administration, to maintain a steady plasma concentration and/or if this is the only route available or tolerated

NB If in doubt always check the British National Formulary (BNF), Summary of product characteristics (SPC), *NHS Injectable Medicines Guide*, or local protocol.

Equipment

- Sharps bin
- Needle (21G green)
- Alcohol wipe
- Gloves
- Diluent
- Drug
- Syringe
- Clean plastic tray
- Prescription
- Vial containing the injectable medicine

Medical Student Survival Skills: Procedural Skills, First Edition. Philip Jevon and Ruchi Joshi.
© 2020 John Wiley & Sons Ltd. Published 2020 by John Wiley & Sons Ltd.
Companion website: www.wiley.com/go/jevon/medicalstudent

Preparation

- Read the prescription details to confirm that they relate to the patient to be treated
- Area in which the drugs are prepared should be clean, uncluttered, and free from distraction
- Use aseptic non-touch technique (ANNT)
- Check all packaging and containers for expiry date and if stored as recommended
- Check the dose, diluent, route of administration, and rate of delivery against the prescription and product information

Cautions and contraindications

- Always use ANNT
- Patient refusal and allergy to the drug to be given

Procedure

- Clean hands
- Wear protective and disposable gloves
- Disinfect the surface of the plastic tray
- Check medicine vial – name of medicine, amount of medicine in the vial, route of administration, and expiry date
- Ask a colleague to cross check the above components
- Check the expiry date, name, and amount and route of the diluent
- Cross check the diluent with a colleague
- Remove the plastic or aluminium cap from the vial
- Clean the rubber septum with an alcohol wipe and leave to dry
- Assemble all needles and syringes and keep them on a tray using ANTT
- Draw up the diluent
  - Twist the plastic top to open the diluent or snap open the neck of a glass ampoule
  - Invert the diluent ampoule
  - Draw up the diluent using needle and syringe
  - Invert the syringe once you have drawn up the diluent, and expel any air by tapping at the end of the syringe

- Add the diluent in to the medicine vial
  - Pierce the rubber septum of the vial with the needle
  - Hold the vial upright
  - Withdraw some air from the vial and add diluent repeatedly until the diluent is in the vial
- Dissolve the medicine in diluent
  - Do not remove the needle when doing this as this can reduce sterility
  - Shake the vial until the powder is dissolved and the solution is clear
- Calculate the volume of solution that contains the required dose
  - It is good practice to cross check the calculated dose
- Withdraw the solution from the vial
  - Invert the vial
  - Suck out 1–2 ml of solution and then push in 1–2 ml of air repeatedly until the required amount of solution is in the syringe
- Expel any trapped air in the syringe
- Discard the needle in the sharps bin
- Label your syringe

Post-procedure checks

- Check the prescription again
- Make sure the calculated dose is correct

OSCE Key Learning Points

✔ Do not discard the vial until you have completed administration to the patient

✔ If you only need 5 ml out of 10 ml solution to administer the required dose to the patient, always discard the rest of the 5 ml of solution from the syringe before you go to the patient

24 Dosage and administration of insulin and use of sliding scales

Introduction

- Insulin is an essential and life-saving medication for thousands of patients who suffer with diabetes. However, it is essential to recognise that it also has the potential to cause severe harm and in some cases death when prescribed or administered incorrectly
- Overdosing a patient with insulin is a *never event* as it can lead to life-threatening hypoglycaemia
- Underdosing a patient also leads to dangerous complications of diabetic ketoacidois (DKA) or a hyperosmolar hyperglycaemic state and is detrimental to long-term glycaemic control

Types of insulin

- Rapid-acting insulin is given with meals. It acts quickly within 20 minutes and can be delivered subcutaneously via injection or a pump. It is more commonly used in type 1 diabetes but is sometimes used in type 2 and it has a higher risk of causing hypoglycaemia. Examples include Humalog and Novorapid
- Long-acting insulin lasts much longer than rapid-acting insulin, it is administered once or twice per day, and is used in both type 1 and 2 diabetes. Although it can also cause hypoglycaemia, the risk is less than in rapid-acting insulin. Examples include Lantus and Levemir

Medical Student Survival Skills: Procedural Skills, First Edition. Philip Jevon and Ruchi Joshi.
© 2020 John Wiley & Sons Ltd. Published 2020 by John Wiley & Sons Ltd.
Companion website: www.wiley.com/go/jevon/medicalstudent

Prescribing insulin

- Always check the patient's normal insulin regime. Ideally this is done when the patient brings in their own medication and is also checked verbally with the patient if this is possible. If it is not possible, other sources include the patient's GP or a recent discharge summary although this should be done with caution
- Most hospitals have a separate drug chart specifically for insulin prescribing; however in some trusts insulin will be prescribed on the standard drug chart. Check your local policy
- Prescribe the insulin on the chart, including the following:
  - Full name of insulin, e.g. Novomix 30
  - The number of units required – units should not be abbreviated to 'U' but should be written in full
  - The route, which will usually be subcutaneous
  - Time of administration
  - Name, signature, and bleep of prescriber
- It is not acceptable to postpone insulin prescribing because the patient is admitted out of hours. If you are unsure about what dose to prescribe discuss with a senior or the diabetic specialist nurse
- Any decision to omit insulin or change an insulin prescription must be done by a qualified doctor who may seek assistance from the diabetes specialist nurses or medical team if required

Administration

- Insulin should only be measured and administered using an insulin syringe or commercial insulin pen
- Staff administering insulin should have had appropriate training
- Always check the name, dose, time, and method of administration before insulin is given

Sliding scales

- The term sliding scale often referred to as Variable Rate Intravenous Insulin Infusions (VRIII) refers to a regime of short-acting insulin dosing that is targeted to predetermined ranges in blood glucose
- The insulin infusion is prepared by adding 50 units of Actrapid insulin to 50 ml of 0.9% saline; therefore 1 ml of the solution contains 1 unit of Actrapid. The goal is to achieve blood glucose control within the range of 5–10 mmol l^{-1}. Blood glucose is measured, at the minimum, on an hourly basis

Indications

Sliding scales are used primarily in three circumstances:
- Treatment of DKA
- Treatment of the hyperosmolar hyperglycaemic state
- Patients who are diabetic and need to be nil by mouth (usually surgical patients)

However, they can also be used when a patient's diabetic control has been disrupted because they are acutely unwell, for example during sepsis.

Setting up a sliding scale insulin regime

- In most hospitals a pre-printed sheet will be provided that will have the dosing regime. This needs to signed and reviewed on a regular basis
- In addition to the insulin infusion you will need to prescribe an appropriate IV fluid regime that will run alongside the insulin infusion. This should usually be given through the same cannula to avoid only one of the regimes being delivered in the event of a blocked cannula
- In patients who are nil by mouth an appropriate regime would be 1 l of 5–10% glucose with 20 mmol of potassium chloride (KCl) over 8 hours
- In patients with disrupted blood glucose control or with DKA/hyperosmolar hyperglycaemic state, an appropriate fluid regime would be 1 l 0.9% saline with 20 mmol KCl over 8 hours, until blood glucose is less than 12 mmol l⁻¹

NB
- If the patient is hypo- or hypervolaemic then the volume or rate of fluid infusion may need to be adjusted
- There is some variation between trusts as to the rate of infusion; be sure to check your local policy
- Discontinue normal insulin and oral antihyperglycaemics unless the patient is being treated for DKA or hyperosmolar hyperglycaemia; in the latter, continue normal regimes

- Venous glucose and urea and electrolytes (U&Es) should be checked on a daily basis
- The regime must be reviewed by a senior at least every 24 hours and the need for sliding scale checked
- A new regime must be prescribed every 24 hours

Stopping a sliding scale

- Patients should not stay on a sliding scale for longer than is clinically necessary
- Prescribe a normal insulin regime on the drug chart
- Long-acting insulin should be started prior to the sliding scale being stopped
- Tight monitoring is essential after stopping the sliding scale
- Poor control after stopping a sliding scale is not an indication to restart

Problems encountered

- If blood glucose is not being controlled by the sliding scale, first check that the cannula is working and the infusion is running appropriately. If no problem is identified then take a venous blood glucose and U&Es for a bicarbonate level and seek senior help. An increase in dose may be required
- If blood glucose is less than 4, check that the glucose infusion is running. If blood glucose is persistently less than 4, increase glucose to 10% and discuss with seniors. Doses may need to be halved
- If blood glucose is less than 2, stop immediately and treat for hypoglycaemia

 NB If you are unsure about prescribing a sliding scale always seek senior help. Most hospitals will have diabetic specialist nurses available via a bleep, they are very skilled and will often be able to help.

Introduction

- A subcutaneous injection is an injection inserting medicine into the fatty vascular layer between the dermis and muscle
- They are used in all age ranges, often for vaccination administration
- Medicines commonly injected subcutaneously include insulin and low molecular weight heparin (LMWH)
- Sites of subcutaneous injection:
  - Arm (biceps)
  - Thigh
  - Abdomen

 NB For repeated injections, regularly change the injection site.

Contraindications

- Allergy to medicine!

Equipment

- 2× blue needles
- Steret
- Syringe appropriate to dose
- Gloves
- Cotton wool
- Sharps bin

Medical Student Survival Skills: Procedural Skills, First Edition. Philip Jevon and Ruchi Joshi.
© 2020 John Wiley & Sons Ltd. Published 2020 by John Wiley & Sons Ltd.
Companion website: www.wiley.com/go/jevon/medicalstudent

Procedure for insertion

Pre-procedure

- Wash hands and don non-sterile gloves
- Prepare equipment.
- Check details of patient's wristband, verbally with patient, drug chart, and medicine in hand.
- Assemble needle to syringe.
- Withdraw correct volume of medicine in syringe
- Change needles
- Explain procedure to the patient

Procedure

- Clean skin
- Pinch skin between two fingers
- Insert needle into skin at 45°.
- Withdraw syringe slightly to ensure no vessels have been hit
- Inject medicine
- Withdraw needle at the same angle that it was inserted
- Have a plaster to hand!

Post-procedure

- First and foremost dispose of sharps safely
- Check patient
- Patient should remain seated in the clinical setting for 1 minute in case of reaction

---

OSCE Key Learning Points

✔ Do not forget to withdraw the syringe slightly before injecting medicine
✔ Never forget safe disposal of sharps

Complications

- Anaphylaxis
- Mild allergic reaction – rash
- Swelling or erythema round injection site
- Cold/flu symptoms (depending on injection)
- Lipodystrophy (chronic)

 Common misinterpretations and pitfalls

It is not an intramuscular injection!

26 Intravenous injections

Introduction

- IV infusions are one of the most common treatments received by patients in hospital
- IV infusions can range from simple maintenance fluids or drugs to emergency transfusions of blood and blood products
- IV infusions are required for:
  - Administering fluids, either as maintenance or replacement
  - Administering drugs to the circulation
  - Administering blood or blood products
- The patient will require IV access in some form, either a peripheral cannula or central venous catheter

Equipment

Giving set

- IV infusions are administered to the patient via a 'giving set'. This is a plastic tube with two specialised ends, a 'spike' which goes to the fluid bag and a 'Luer lock' connector for attachment to the IV access route
- The connections on fluid bags and IV access methods are standardised in the UK
- The giving set typically has two chambers to allow for visualisation of fluid flow and to prevent air infiltrating from the bag. The giving set also has a flow control wheel that compresses the plastic tubing allowing for crude control over the rate of infusion

Fluid bag

- Fluid bags typically have two ports on their underside: an injection port, which is soft and spongy allowing for additives to be injected into the bag, and a port for the 'spike' of the giving set

Medical Student Survival Skills: Procedural Skills, First Edition. Philip Jevon and Ruchi Joshi.
© 2020 John Wiley & Sons Ltd. Published 2020 by John Wiley & Sons Ltd.
Companion website: www.wiley.com/go/jevon/medicalstudent

Other equipment

- Correctly prescribed bag of fluid/pre-prepared drug for infusion/blood product
- Chlorhexidine 2% wipe
- Non-sterile gloves
- Apron
- Tray to transport infusion to patient

Procedure for IV infusion

Pre-procedure

- Inform the patient that they are to receive IV therapy, and the duration of time they will be connected to the infusion
- Gain consent for the procedure
- Set up a sterile field onto a trolley
- Don an apron and non-sterile gloves. This clinical skill may be carried out in a ward preparation room and does not need to be done at the bedside. You will need a colleague to check the infusion with
- Before you begin, observe the bag of fluid for any particulate matter, leaking, or cloudiness. If any are seen, the bag must be discarded and reported to the manufacturer. Once you are satisfied with the fluid, check the prescription with your colleague and document that a two person check has taken place

Procedure

- Remove the packaging from the bag of fluid and giving set
- Move the infusion control wheel to completely occlude the tubing ('off position')
- Snap off the port from the fluid bag (adjacent to the injection port)
- Remove the cover from the giving set spike. Take care not to touch it once the cover is removed. If you do, you must discard the giving set as it is contaminated
- With the bag of fluid upside down, firmly push the spike through the port. A twisting motion may help (Figure 26.1)
- With the bag still upside down, squeeze it gently to expel any air down the non-primed line. This will reduce the risk of air infiltrating the line when the bag of fluid is empty
- Squeeze the upper chamber of the giving set to half fill it

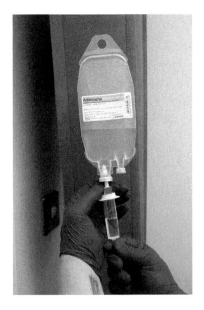

Figure 26.1 Connecting the giving set to the IV fluid bag.

- Direct the Luer lock end of the giving set to waste. Hold the bag of fluid up and minimally open the flow control wheel. Fluid will begin to rush down the tubing and out of the Luer lock end. Ensure that no air bubbles are seen in the tube and the fluid runs smoothly
- Close the infusion control wheel once again
- Place the primed infusion into a tray/trolley and take it to the patient
- Check the following before connecting the infusion:
  - *Correct patient*
    - Name and date of birth, hospital number, and address (check the wristband)
    - Allergy status
  - *Correct prescription*
    - Right fluid
    - Right volume
  - *Correct date and time*
  - *Correct infusion rate*
- Remove the cap from the IV access route and dispose
- Clean with 2% chlorhexine wipe or equivalent and allow to dry
- Connect infusion to patient. Twist the Luer connector to lock it to the patient
- Open the flow control wheel to the desired rate

Cautions

- IV fluids are commonly poorly prescribed. It is important to determine the fluid balance of a patient before commencing IV fluids
- Certain medications must be given via specific IV routes. Consult the summary of product characteristics (SPC) of a drug for further information
- Air must *not* be allowed to infiltrate down the line into the patient. Carefully inspect the line for air bubbles

Common problems

- Air in the line – commonly caused by allowing air to infiltrate from the bag. Opening the line to allow air to be flushed out works well. Flicking the line to dislodge air bubbles with the control wheel open also works well. If air persists and cannot be removed, the line and fluid bag must be discarded
- Fluid not infusing – ensure that the control wheel is not in the off position. Ensure the line is not kinked. Observe the site of IV access for patency. It may be necessary to flush the peripheral cannula to open a valve or unkink the lumen to allow for free-flowing infusion

27 Administration of blood transfusion

Introduction

- Blood transfusion is an essential and significant part of modern healthcare treatment
- The process of blood transfusion requires careful preparation and treatment to minimise risks and complications
- Most importantly, a patient receiving a transfusion of blood products must be adequately monitored so that any adverse reactions/complications can be recognised promptly and effectively treated and managed

Blood components and their uses

When the National Blood Service centrifuges whole donor blood it then can be separated and processed into blood components for transfusion:

- Red cells (erythrocytes)
- White blood cells (granulocytes/leucocytes)
- Platelets (thrombocytes)
- Plasma (contains clotting factors)

NB All blood donations are tested to detect human immunodeficiency virus (HIV), hepatitis B, hepatitis C, syphilis and human T-cell leukaemia virus (HTLV).

Red cells

- Once the plasma and buffy coat (white blood cell and platelets) have been removed from whole blood the red cells are suspended in an additive solution for preservation purposes during storage

Medical Student Survival Skills: Procedural Skills, First Edition. Philip Jevon and Ruchi Joshi.
© 2020 John Wiley & Sons Ltd. Published 2020 by John Wiley & Sons Ltd.
Companion website: www.wiley.com/go/jevon/medicalstudent

- Red cells are stored at 2–6 °C in a temperature controlled fridge and have a shelf life of 35 days from the date of donation
- Once collected from blood storage, red cells should be transfused within 4 hours
- The decision to transfuse red cells is a complex one and depends on factors such as cause of anaemia, severity, the patient's ability to compensate for the anaemia, and the likelihood of further blood loss

OSCE Key Learning Points ⊕

Red cell compatibility

Patient blood group	Red cell antigens	Plasma antibodies	Donor group compatibility
A	A	Anti-B	A and O
B	B	Anti-A	B and O
AB	AB	None	A, B, AB, and O
O	O	Anti-A and anti-B	O

Fresh frozen plasma (FFP)

- Standard FFP is frozen and stored at −30 °C with a shelf life of 24 months. If required, FFP is rapidly thawed at 37 °C before being issued
- Once thawed, FFP should be transfused within 4 hours (if FFP is stored at 4 °C post-thawing, the transfusion must be completed within 24 hours)
- FFP may be indicated if the patient has a single factor deficiency for which there is no virus-safe fractioned product, severe bleeding, disseminated intravascular coagulation (DIC), or thrombotic thrombocytopenic purpura (TTP)
- Table 27.1 shows the principles of selection of FFP

Table 27.1 Selection of FFP according to recipient blood group

Recipient group	O	A	B	AB
1st choice	O	A	B	AB
2nd choice	A	AB	AB	A
3rd choice	B	B	A	B
4th choice	AB			

Cryoprecipitate

- Cryoprecipitate is a plasma product that contains clotting factors such as factor VIII, fibrinogen, and factor XIII
- Its most common use is to enhance fibrinogen levels in dysfibrinogenaemia and acquired hypofibrinogenaemia seen in massive transfusion and DIC
- Treatment is usually indicated if the plasma fibrinogen is less than $1\,gl^{-1}$
- Cryoprecipitate once thawed should be transfused immediately

NB The use of FFP and cryoprecipitate should be guided by monitoring, using laboratory coagulation screens.

Platelets

- All platelets must be stored on a special agitator rack at 20–24 °C to prevent clumping
- Each unit of platelets has a shelf life of 5 days from the date of donation
- Platelet transfusions are indicated for the prevention and treatment of haemorrhage in patients with thrombocytopenia (low platelet count) or platelet function defects. The cause of thrombocytopenia should be established before a decision is made for a platelet transfusion
- Risks associated with platelet transfusions include alloimmunisation, transmission of infection, allergic reactions, and transfusion-related lung injury

Patient identification

 Common misinterpretations and pitfalls

If the patient identification band is missing, defaced, or hidden, this is a significant contributory factor in incidents where the wrong blood is given.

- All patients receiving a blood transfusion must wear a patient identification band; minimum patient identifiers are last name, first name, date of birth, and unique patient identification number. The information must be legible and accurate
- In emergency situations the patient's core identifiers may be unknown; at least one unique identifier, usually a temporary identification number (e.g. accident and emergency number) and the patient's gender must be used

- Patient identification should be checked and confirmed as correct at each stage of the transfusion process. Whenever possible, the patient should be asked to state their full name and date of birth. This must match exactly the information on the patient's wristband and any other associated paperwork required at that stage of the blood transfusion process
- If there are patient identification discrepancies at any stage of the transfusion process, the information must be verified and discrepancies investigated and corrected before proceeding to the next stage of the process

Documentation

Pre-transfusion

- Clinical indication for transfusion
- Pre-transfusion indices (e.g. full blood count, coagulation screen)
- Date of decision
- Date of transfusion
- Blood component to be transfused, and volume
- Rate of transfusion
- Consent from patient
- Special requirements (e.g. irradiated or cytomegalovirus-seronegative components)

Administration

- Date and time component was collected
- Date and time transfusion was commenced
- Donation number of the component transfused
- Volume administered
- Identification of staff who commenced transfusion
- Observations before, during, and after transfusion

Post-transfusion

- Date and time component was completed
- An indication of whether transfusion achieved desired effect
- Outcome of any reactions

Traceability

- All blood components should be traceable from the donor to its final destination, whether this is a recipient, manufacturer, or disposal

- All organisations have a policy on how to achieve this by using electronic or manual methods
- This information is then kept for 30 years

Equipment

Intravenous access

- All blood components can be administered through standard peripheral IV cannulas according to the manufacturer's specifications
- The size of the IV cannula depends on the size and integrity of the vein as well as the speed at which the blood component is to be transfused. All blood components can be slowly infused through a small-bore cannula, e.g. 21G. For a more rapid infusion, a large-bore needle, e.g. 14G, is needed
- Multilumen central lines are usually suitable for transfusion of blood components, although one lumen should be reserved for administering blood components where possible

Administration set

- Blood components must only be administered using a blood administration set that has an integral 170–200 µm screen filter
- It is unnecessary to prime the blood administration set with saline
- The blood administration set should be changed at least every 12 hours and after completion of the prescribed blood transfusion to prevent bacterial growth

NB Platelets should not be transfused through an administration set that has been previously used for red cells or other components as this may cause aggregation and retention of platelets in the line.

Blood warmers

- Rapid infusion of red cells soon after their removal from blood storage refrigeration at 4 °C can lead to hypothermia, arrhythmias, cardiac arrest, or impaired blood clotting in surgical or trauma patients
- Transfused blood components should be warmed to 37 °C in adults undergoing surgery and in patients with clinically significant antibodies

NB Blood must never be warmed in an uncontrolled way, e.g. in a microwave, in hot water, or on a radiator.

Monitoring priorities in a patient receiving a blood transfusion

Pre-transfusion

Baseline observations of temperature, pulse rate, blood pressure, and respiration rate should be taken within 60 minutes before the start of the transfusion.

During transfusion

NB Most serious reactions occur within 30 minutes of commencement of the transfusion of blood component units.

Observations of pulse rate, blood pressure, temperature, and respiration rate should be taken and recorded 15 minutes after commencement of each component transfusion.

Signs of a possible reaction include:

- Pyrexia
- Tachycardia
- Change in blood pressure
- Breathlessness or rapid breathing
- Coughing
- Haemoglobinuria
- Nausea
- Vomiting
- Diarrhoea
- Skin flushing/rash
- Rigors
- Collapse
- Chest, abdominal, bone, muscle, or loin pain
- Headache
- Restlessness, agitation, or confusion

Post-transfusion

- Measure the pulse rate, blood pressure, temperature, and respiratory rate
- Patients should ideally be observed during the subsequent 24 hours

Adverse reactions to blood transfusion

- Acute haemolytic transfusion reaction
- Infusion of a bacterially contaminated unit
- Transfusion-related acute lung injury (TRALI)
- Severe allergic reaction or anaphylaxis
- Post-transfusion Purpura (PTP)
- Transfusion-associated graft versus host disease

NB In all cases, expert medical advice can be sought from a haematologist and the blood transfusion department must be informed as soon as possible. This department may need to inform the National Blood Service or the Medicines and Healthcare Products Regulatory Agency.

28 Male and female urinary catheterisation

Introduction

- This is common procedure that needs to be performed correctly with particular attention to aseptic technique
- Maintaining the patient's dignity and privacy is paramount

Indications

- Acute urinary retention, e.g. acute bladder outlet obstruction
- Monitoring fluid balance in critically ill patients, e.g. sepsis
- Maintaining a continuous outflow of urine for patients with voiding difficulties, as a result of neurological disorders that cause paralysis or loss of sensation affecting urination
- Anticipated prolonged duration of surgery
- Management of intractable incontinence
- To improve comfort for end of life
- Instillation of drugs into bladder, e.g. chemotherapy agents

Types of catheters

- Standard two way catheters (Figure 28.1)
- Three way catheters – for patients presenting with macroscopic haematuria or clot retention where irrigation can be used through the extra port to wash out the bladder
- Tiemann catheter – these have a pointed tip and can be used to negotiate the curve in the male prostatic urethra and can be helpful for difficult insertions

Medical Student Survival Skills: Procedural Skills, First Edition. Philip Jevon and Ruchi Joshi.
© 2020 John Wiley & Sons Ltd. Published 2020 by John Wiley & Sons Ltd.
Companion website: www.wiley.com/go/jevon/medicalstudent

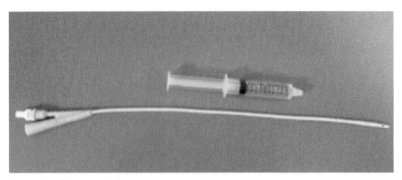

Figure 28.1 Two way catheter.

Procedure for male urinary catheterisation

Introduction and consent

- Identify the patient and introduce yourself. Inform them why a catheter is needed whilst obtaining their consent for the procedure
- A chaperone should be present who can also assist you

Equipment (Figure 28.2)

- Catheterisation pack – this should include a sterile drape, swabs, gauze, collecting tray, and pot
- A size 14Fr male Foley catheter to begin with

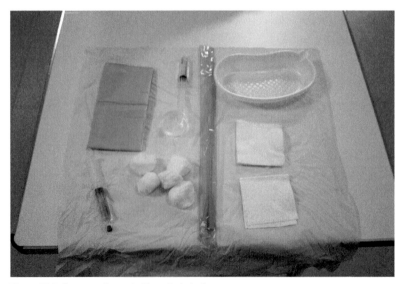

Figure 28.2 Components needed for catheterisation.

- Sterile gloves – you can either use two pairs of gloves (de-glove one pair during the procedure) or use the clean hand/dirty hand technique using one pair of gloves (in the procedure section we will discuss the two pair glove technique)
- Lignocaine anaesthetic gel (to anaesthetise, disinfect, and lubricate the urethra)
- Antiseptic solution
- A 10 ml saline pre-filled syringe (normally comes with the catheter)
- Catheter bag
- A clean two-tier trolley

Positioning

- Position the patient supine, with legs apart (Figure 28.3)

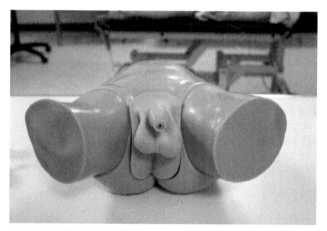

Figure 28.3 Mannequin model portraying correct positioning for a male patient.

 NB Always have a chaperone.

Preparation

- Wash and dry hands thoroughly.
- Place the catheterisation pack on top of the trolley, opening it whilst not touching the sterile field inside, i.e. aseptic (no-touch) technique.
- Pour the antiseptic solution into the pot.
- Open and place the catheter, 10 ml pre-filled saline syringe, and lignocaine anaesthetic gel onto the sterile field aseptically.

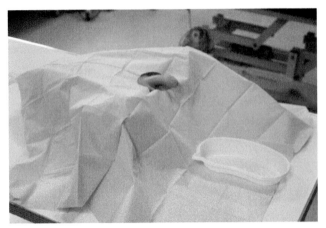

Figure 28.4 Sterile drape placed correctly over patient with collecting tray as shown.

- Place the sterile drape over the patient with the collecting tray in between the patient's legs (Figure 28.4)
- Put on your two pairs of sterile gloves

Procedure
- Hold the penis with a sterile gauze with one hand (if applicable retract the foreskin) and clean thoroughly using the antiseptic solution-soaked swab around the urethral meatus with the non-dominant hand (Figure 28.5).

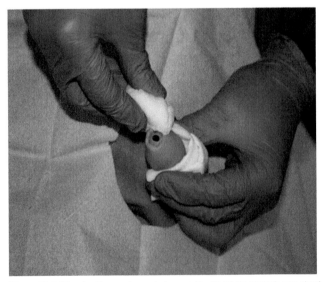

Figure 28.5 Cleaning the meatus and glans penis with sterile gauze in non-dominant hand.

Repeat at least three times, starting with the meatus and work your way outwards when cleaning the glans penis

- Using the lignocaine anaesthetic gel, apply a tiny amount (approximately 1 ml) around the meatus (Figure 28.6) and then insert the tip of the syringe into the opening of the meatus injecting the remaining lignocaine gel into the urethra at a steady slow rate (Figure 28.7). Hold the lignocaine syringe against the meatus for at least 30 seconds to prevent the gel seeping out
- The anaesthetic gel should ideally be given 5 minutes to take effect
- At this point de-glove one pair of used sterile gloves (Figure 28.8)
- Carefully position the tip of the catheter into the urethra (Figure 28.9)

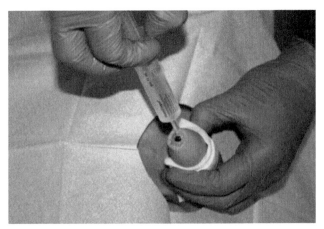

Figure 28.6 Anaesthetic gel being applied around the meatus.

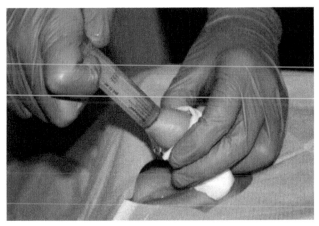

Figure 28.7 Anaesthetic gel being inserted into the urethra via meatus.

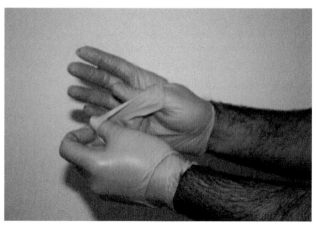

Figure 28.8 De-gloving first pair of used sterile gloves.

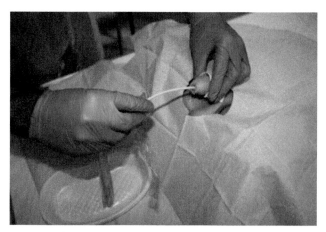

Figure 28.9 Penis held at 90° to the vertical whilst inserting the catheter initially.

- Upon catheter insertion, use the non-dominant hand to maintain the penis taut when initially advancing the catheter into the urethra
- Avoid contact between your advancing hand and the meatus
- Advance the catheter while holding the penis in a vertical position to help straighten the urethra (Figure 28.10)
- If resistance is felt then asking the patient to arch their back or coughing whilst you advance the catheter are useful techniques to aid progress into the bladder (this alleviates perineal muscle spasm). In addition using more anaesthetic gel may help

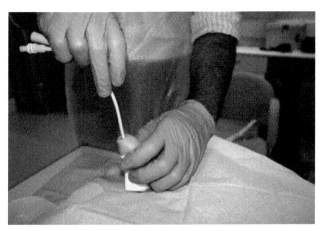

Figure 28.10 Ensure penis is held at 90° while advancing catheter.

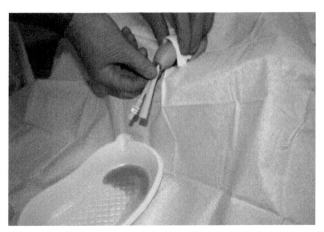

Figure 28.11 Catheter being inserted until the hilt of the catheter is in contact with the meatus.

- When the catheter tip is in the bladder, urine should begin to flow from the catheter into the collecting tray. Ensure the catheter hilt touches the meatus (Figure 28.11)
- Once urine flow is seen and the catheter has been fully inserted, inflate the catheter balloon slowly with the pre-filled saline syringe (Figure 28.12), assessing for acute pain. All catheter packaging will state how much volume is needed to inflate the balloon
- The catheter should then be pulled back until resistance is felt to ensure the catheter is secure and the balloon is sitting just above the bladder neck (Figure 28.13)

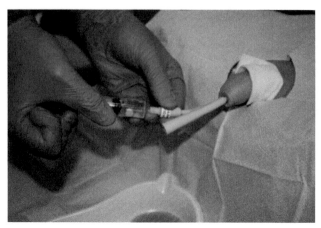

Figure 28.12 Urine flow prompts inflation of catheter balloon using the pre-filled saline syringe.

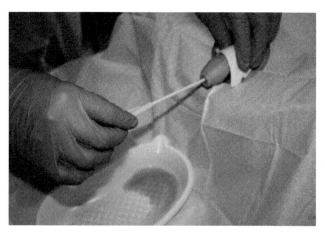

Figure 28.13 Pulling back on catheter confirming catheter balloon position above bladder neck.

- Retracting the foreskin is crucial. If forgotten this will put the patient at risk of developing paraphimosis
- Attach the catheter bag to the catheter so the residual volume can be measured (Figure 28.14)

Post-procedure
- Dispose gloves and equipment into a clinical waste bin *except* for the catheter labels found on the packaging, which will be needed for documentation purposes.
- Thank the patient and ask them to cover up.

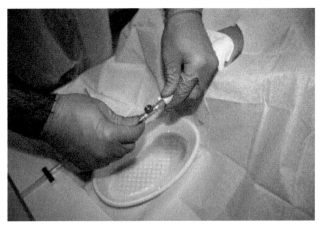

Figure 28.14 Catheter bag being attached to catheter port.

- Wash your hands.
- Document the procedure. A summary of the procedure should be documented explaining: the indication, the use of aseptic technique, catheter size (via labels), ease of catheter insertion, volume used to inflate the catheter balloon, foreskin retraction (if applicable), and residual volume drained
- A urine sample should ideally be sent for microscopy, culture, and sensitivity
- Consult local guidelines if antibiotic prophylaxis is required to prevent catheter-associated urinary tract infections – it is routinely given for traumatic catheterisations or for a change of catheter.

Procedure for female urinary catheterisation

Positioning

- Always have a chaperone
- Instruct the patient to lie supine with legs apart as good exposure is important

Preparation

- Wash and dry hands thoroughly
- Place the catheterisation pack on top of the trolley, opening it whilst not touching the sterile field inside, i.e. aseptic (no-touch) technique
- Pour the antiseptic solution into the pot.
- Open and place the catheter, 10 ml pre-filled saline syringe, and lignocaine anaesthetic gel onto the sterile field aseptically.

- Place the sterile drape over the patient with the collecting tray in between the patient's legs
- In this instance one pair of sterile gloves may be used
- Clean around the labia minora and urethral opening with antiseptic solution (Figures 28.15 and 28.16)
- Place lignocaine anaesthetic gel into the urethra and onto the catheter

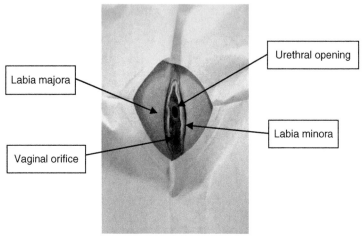

Urethral opening

Labia majora

Labia minora

Vaginal orifice

Figure 28.15 External anatomy of female urogenital area.

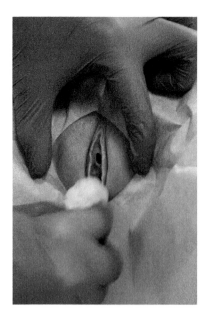

Figure 28.16 Cleaning the urethral opening and surroundings with antiseptic solution.

Procedure

- Holding the catheter by its sleeve, use the non-dominant hand to keep the labia minora apart, advancing the catheter into the urethra until urine flow is seen (Figure 28.17)
- Once urine flow is seen (Figure 28.18), inflate the catheter balloon. All catheter packaging will state how much volume is needed to inflate the balloon
- Attach the catheter bag to measure the residual volume

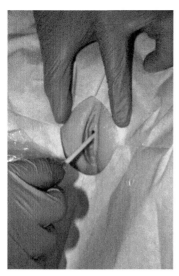
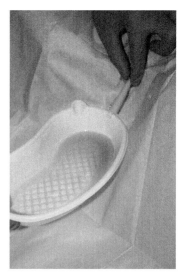

Figure 28.17 Catheter insertion into urethral orifice.

Figure 28.18 Urine flow achieved indicating catheter tip is in bladder.

Post-procedure

- Dispose gloves and equipment into a clinical waste bin *except* for the catheter labels found on the packaging, which will be needed for documentation purposes.
- Thank the patient and ask them to cover up.
- Wash your hands.
- Document the procedure. A summary of the procedure should be documented explaining: the indication, the use of aseptic technique, ease of catheter insertion, volume used to inflate the catheter balloon, residual volume, and catheter size (via labels)
- Send a urine sample for microscopy, culture, and sensitivity
- Consult local guidelines if antibiotic prophylaxis is required to prevent catheter-associated urinary tract infections – it is routinely given for traumatic catheterisations or for a change of catheter

29 Instructing patients in the use of devices for inhaled medication

Introduction

- An inhaler is a medical device that allows the administration of drugs via the lungs
- It means drugs can be given at a much lower dose than if given orally, leading to reduced side effects
- There are many different types of inhalation devices. Their use will vary, depending on the patient's age, medical history, and preference.
- The anatomy of the airways ensures that large particles are filtered out before reaching the lungs
- Smaller particles can be delivered straight to the airways via inhalation devices, when delivered at the correct speed and with the correct inhaler technique
- Incorrect inhaler technique is more likely in children or in older and more debilitated patients, who may have poor coordination; this can lead to poor disease control and affect the overall prognosis of the patient, including poor quality of life and an increase in hospital admissions

Types of inhaler device

- MDI – metered dose inhaler
- BA-MDI – breath activated metered dose inhaler
- DPI – dry powder inhaler

Medical Student Survival Skills: Procedural Skills, First Edition. Philip Jevon and Ruchi Joshi.
© 2020 John Wiley & Sons Ltd. Published 2020 by John Wiley & Sons Ltd.
Companion website: www.wiley.com/go/jevon/medicalstudent

Indications

Acute bronchoconstriction

- This requires use of a short-acting bronchodilator
- A bronchodilator is also known as a 'reliever' inhaler, for example salbutamol and terbutaline

Prevention of bronchoconstriction

- Here, inhalers are taken every day to prevent symptoms of bronchoconstriction
- A steroid is usually required, this reduces the inflammation in the airways and therefore reduces the risk of airway constriction
- Bronchodilators can also contain long-acting beta-agonists to further control symptoms

 Common misinterpretations and pitfalls

Poor inhaler technique can often be mistaken for poor response to treatment – always review inhaler technique!

Equipment

- Inhaler
- Spacer

Procedure for instructing patients in the use of devices for inhaled medication

Pre-procedure

- Identify correct medication
- Identify correct patient
- Explain procedure to the patient
- Wash hands

Procedure

- Remove the cap, shake well, and hold the inhaler upright
- Take a gentle breath out and hold
- Insert the mouth piece of the inhaler into the mouth and close teeth around this gently. Form a tight seal with the lips

- Take a long slow breath in and press the canister as firmly as you can do so
- Hold your breath for 10 seconds or for as long as is comfortable
- Remove the inhaler from the mouth
- Breathe out gently
- For a second dose, wait 1 minute and then repeat previous steps

Post-procedure
- Replace cap

NB
- Use of steroid inhalers may cause oral candidiasis and a hoarse voice
- This is due to deposition of the steroid at the oropharynx, which may be caused by incorrect inhaler technique
- This can be avoided by brushing the teeth after taking the inhaler or through the use of a spacer device

Use of a spacer device

- A spacer is a device that can be used with an MDI inhaler
- It holds the medication released from the inhaler like a reservoir
- It has a valve that opens when the patient breathes in. This allows inhalation of the medication in but prevents it from escaping back into the spacer
- It also reduces the speed of the medication particles, reducing the amount deposited at the oropharynx
- Spacers are useful for those patients with poor coordination, in children, and in those prone to oral candidiasis

OSCE Key Learning Points

Signs of a severe asthma attack
- ✓ Respiratory rate >25 min^{-1}
- ✓ Pulse >110 min^{-1}
- ✓ Difficulty in completing sentences in one breath

30 Skin suturing

Miranvir Singh Jaspal

Leicester University, Leicester, UK

Introduction

- It is important to use the correct suture and technique in order to close a wound appropriately to prevent infection, wound damage, and to stop bleeding
- Lacerations can be caused by different mechanisms and involve different sites that dictate the method used before suturing
- It is important to maintain haemostasis through direct pressure or elevation but if severe a tourniquet or clamp/suture may be required for arterial bleeds

Pre-procedure considerations

- *Clean wounds* – these are wounds that are caused by uncontaminated objects, generally sharp, which can be in one piece or broken, e.g. glass
- *Contaminated/dirty wounds* – these are wounds that are caused by contaminated objects, containing soil, dirt, rust, faecal/bowel matter, etc. – these will need thorough irrigation, cleaning, and antibiotic cover
- *Impact* – the mechanism of impact is vital as it allows assessment of the wound and especially of the underlying structures such as the tendons, nerves, ligaments, and bone. These structures may need to be attended to (by specialist teams – orthopaedic/plastic surgeons) if damaged before the repair of the superficial wound
- *X-rays* – these may be of help in penetrating injuries to identify deep damage or if retained objects are present – this may dictate if the wound needs exploration
- *Delayed healing* – this may occur in older age groups, and those with diabetes, infected wounds, ischaemia, nutrition deficiency, smoking, steroid therapy, foreign bodies, and connective tissue disorders

Medical Student Survival Skills: Procedural Skills, First Edition. Philip Jevon and Ruchi Joshi.
© 2020 John Wiley & Sons Ltd. Published 2020 by John Wiley & Sons Ltd.
Companion website: www.wiley.com/go/jevon/medicalstudent

Indications

- Clean, low risk of infection
- Edges can be opposed
- No underlying neurovascular damage
- No underlying muscle or tendon damage

Cautions

- Simple wounds should be closed immediately if < 12 hours old (24 hours for the face)
- Do delayed closure if there is a high risk of infection, give prophylactic antibiotics, and close if there is no infection after about 4 days
- Be careful with jagged edges/underlying structure damage

Relative contraindications

- Infected wound
- Inflamed wound
- Bite wounds: human or animal
- Contaminated by soil/faeces
- Serious crush wounds

 NB Always ask your senior or consult the appropriate specialist if you have concerns about the wound – what appears a simple wound could be limb- or life-threatening.

Equipment

- Suture material: 6.0 nylon – face, 5.0 nylon – on a child anywhere else, 4.0 nylon – hand, 3.0 nylon or silk – scalp/arm/abdomen/trunk, 3.0 nylon – leg
- Absorbable sutures – Vicryl, catgut, polydioxanone, Dexon
- Non-absorbable sutures – nylon, prolene, silk
- Suture kit – needle holder, forceps (toothed, non-toothed), scissors, clean sheet, gauze
- Normal saline irrigation kit
- 1% lidocaine anaesthetic for injection, 10 ml syringe, blue needle
- Steristrips and wound cover adhesive

Procedure for suturing

- Give 1% lidocaine injection to the surrounding wound edges
- Start at one end – go through one surface 5 mm from the wound edge, with the needle 90° to the entry point
- Curve the motion of the forceps in the hand *not* with a pushing motion – this allows gliding of the suture needle and hence less tissue damage
- The needle exits half of the wound and is picked up by the needle holder
- The needle holder transfers the needle to the forceps for repositioning
- Enter the wound with a curved motion until the needle pierces the healthy skin 5 mm from the wound edge
- Triple loop the needle-side suture around the forceps and pull the distal end through
- Lay the knot flat and neat
- Double loop the needle-side suture around the forceps and pull the distal end through
- Lay the knot flat and neat
- Single loop the needle-side suture around the forceps and pull the distal end through
- Lay the knot flat and neat
- Use the forceps to pull the knot to lie lateral to the wound *not* above it
- Cut the ends leaving enough for the nurse to remove the sutures after 5 days, e.g. 3–5 mm
- Repeat until the wound edges are closed
- Leave a gap of 5–10 mm between each suture
- Applied steristrips over the wound to help opposition and dress the wound
- Give antibiotics as appropriate
- Inform the patient if the sutures need to be removed in 5–7 days by the GP nurse

OSCE Key Learning Points

✔ Entry and exit points should be 5 mm from the wound edge and also 5 mm apart from each other
✔ Oppose the wound edges together

Complications

- Containing the infection – the patient may return with a discharging/painful/infected wound
- Skin tearing – if the sutures are applied too tightly
- Poor wound healing – if the sutures are too loose, or an underlying disorder is preventing healing
- Scar formation – if a poor surgical technique/sutures were used, or sutures are not removed

 Common misinterpretations and pitfalls

A simple wound may be misleading and have deep structure damage that may require specialist input.

Introduction

- A sling, sometimes referred to as a triangular bandage, is a hanging bandage for the support of an injured or diseased upper limb. It can provide immobolisation and pain relief, although it is only effective if the casualty is sitting up

Types of slings

There are two main types of sling:
- Broad arm sling (sometimes referred to as an arm sling)
- Elevation sling (sometimes referred to as a high arm sling)

Broad arm sling

- This is used to support an injured upper limb in a horizontal or a slightly raised position and to immobolise the arm if there is a chest injury. This position provides the necessary support whilst elevating the affected limb to reduce any existing swelling and preventing any further swelling
- Indications for using a broad arm sling include fractures of the clavicle and wrist and soft tissue injuries to the hand, wrist, forearm, elbow, upper arm, shoulder, scapula, or clavicle

Elevation sling

- Modified version of the arm sling that supports the forearm and hand in a raised position
- Indications for its use include fractures in the hand and soft tissue injuries or cellulites of the hand and fingers
- It can be used to elevate an injured arm or hand to control haemorrhage from wounds in the forearm or hand, to minimise swelling in burn injuries, and to support the chest in complicated rib fractures

Medical Student Survival Skills: Procedural Skills, First Edition. Philip Jevon and Ruchi Joshi.
© 2020 John Wiley & Sons Ltd. Published 2020 by John Wiley & Sons Ltd.
Companion website: www.wiley.com/go/jevon/medicalstudent

'Collar and cuff' sling

- This is a piece of foam covered with a fine netting and is applied in a figure of eight around the casualty's neck and the affected wrist. Although its use is limited, because it does not support the elbow or forearm, it is recommended if the casualty has a fractured humerus

 Common misinterpretations and pitfalls

Leaving jewellery, e.g. rings, on the injured limb can lead to circulatory problems if swelling develops.

Procedure for the application of a broad arm sling

- Ask the casualty to sit down and support their injured limb with the hand of the uninjured side
- Prepare the equipment: triangular bandage, scissors, and tape
- Explain the procedure to the casualty
- If necessary, remove any rings or jewellery from the injured limb (if swelling develops a ring can act as a tourniquet impeding peripheral circulation)
- Place the triangular bandage against the casualty's chest underneath the injured limb; the long edge should be parallel to the sternum, with the upper tip over the casualty's shoulder (Figure 31.1)
- Move the lower tip of the bandage up to meet the upper tip at the shoulder and tie the two tips together using a reef knot (Figure 31.2)
- Ask the casualty to stop supporting the injured limb
- Fold in the bandage at the elbow and secure with tape (or a safety pin); if these are not available, twist the point of the bandage up until it slots in snugly behind the elbow or back of the arm)
- Monitor the circulation in the injured limb, e.g. pulse, colour, sensation, and temperature; if necessary loosen or reapply

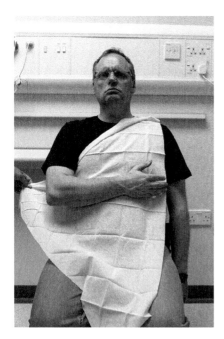

Figure 31.1 Broad arm sling: place the triangular bandage against the casualty's chest.

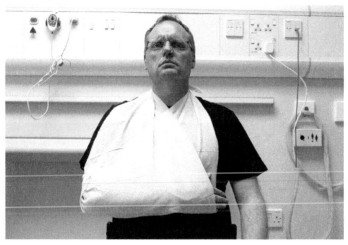

Figure 31.2 Broad arm sling: move the lower tip of the bandage up to meet the upper tip at the shoulder and tie the two tips together using a reef knot.

Procedure for the application of an elevation sling

- Ask the casualty to sit down and support the injured limb across their chest: the fingers of the injured limb should be touching the clavicle of the uninjured side
- Prepare the equipment: triangular bandage, scissors, and tape
- Explain the procedure to the casualty
- If necessary, remove any rings or jewellery from the injured limb
- Place the triangular bandage against the casualty's chest over the injured limb; the long edge should be parallel to the sternum, with the upper tip over the casualty's shoulder
- Move the lower tip of the bandage up to the elbow and while asking the casualty to let go of the injured limb, tuck the tip of the bandage underneath it taking it through to their back
- Tie the two tips together using a reef knot
- Fold in the bandage at the elbow and secure with tape
- Monitor the circulation in the injured limb, e.g. pulse, colour, sensation, and temperature; if necessary loosen or reapply
- Arrange referral to appropriate medical help

Improvised slings

- In the first aid setting, if a bandage is not available, an improvised sling using the casualty's clothing or a belt can be just as effective

---

OSCE Key Learning Points

✔ Remember the patient will probably be in pain
✔ Monitor the circulation in the injured limb, e.g. pulse, colour, sensation, and temperature; if necessary loosen or reapply

Safe disposal of clinical waste, needles, and other 'sharps'

Introduction

- Safe disposal of clinical waste limits transmission of disease
- Safe disposal of sharps limits injury and the spread of blood-borne diseases (e.g. human immunodeficiency virus (HIV), hepatitis)
- Knowledge or safe disposal of sharps and clinical waste is mandatory for anyone working in a healthcare environment
- Any disposable item that has been in contact with a patient, or a patient's bodily fluids, is considered 'clinical waste'
- Any item that has the potential to pierce or cut the skin (e.g. needles, opened glass ampoules, broken crockery) is considered a 'sharp'
- Safe disposal of sharps and clinical waste is the responsibility of the person performing the procedure
- Correct disposal of clinical waste and sharps inspires your patients' confidence

Indications

Types of sharps

- A sharp is anything that has the potential to pierce or cut skin: the following lists are examples and are not. If in doubt, ask
- 'Clean' sharps have not been in contact with bodily fluids. For example:
  - Needles used to draw up drugs
  - Glass ampoules of drugs

Medical Student Survival Skills: Procedural Skills, First Edition. Philip Jevon and Ruchi Joshi.
© 2020 John Wiley & Sons Ltd. Published 2020 by John Wiley & Sons Ltd.
Companion website: www.wiley.com/go/jevon/medicalstudent

- 'Dirty' sharps have been in contact with bodily fluids. For example:
  - Needles used to take blood
  - Needles used for injections
  - Cannulas (including the plastic part) that have been used
  - Lumbar puncture needles
  - Suturing needles
  - Guidewire from a nasogastric tube
- Some instruments (e.g. forceps) can be sterilised. Some should be disposed of as sharps. Before you start a procedure, find out how you should deal with the dirty instruments
- Some sharps have been in contact with cytotoxic or radioactive drugs. These have to be handled and disposed of differently. As a medical student, you should not be responsible for this: ask for help

NB: All sharps should always be handled and treated as if they were dirty.

Types of clinical waste

- Clinical waste should always be handled as though it is infectious
- Clinical waste which has been in contact with cytotoxic or radioactive drugs has to handled and disposed of differently. As a medical student, you should not be responsible for this: ask for help

Cautions

- Different institutions use different sharps bins and colour codes: familiarise yourself with local equipment

Contraindications

- Cytotoxic or radioactive waste: you should not handle these materials

Equipment

- Bedside sharps bin
- Procedure tray or trolley

- Clinical waste bag (yellow)
- Gloves
- Apron
- Sharps/equipment necessary for procedure

Procedure for insertion

Pre-procedure

- Obtain informed consent appropriate for procedure (may be verbal or written)
- Prepare equipment, including the equipment listed above
- Identify correct patient
- Introduce yourself to the patient and check that they still consent to the procedure
- Set up a yellow clinical waste bag and a sharps bin
- Position the patient and clean the skin if appropriate
- Unwrap the equipment for the procedure, using a sterile technique if necessary
- Don your personal protective equipment (gloves, apron, face mask, eye shield)
- It is good practice to count the number of sharps you have opened

Procedure

- Perform the procedure as indicated
- If the patient withdraws consent, abandon the procedure when it is possible to do so safely
- Dispose of your sharps in the sharps bin immediately after using them. For example, after withdrawing the needle from a cannula, put it straight into the sharps bin. Do not put it into a procedure tray
- It is good practice to avoid crossing your hands over when you are holding sharps. This reduces the likelihood of you injuring your other hand with the sharp
- If there are other people near you, or near the sharps bin, you must warn them that you are holding a sharp. This is essential if their back is turned. Saying 'sharp behind you' helps to avoid accidents
- Clinical waste should be put straight into a yellow clinical waste bag. Putting it onto any other surface (e.g. bed or table) contaminates that surface and increases the risk of infection

Post-procedure

- Do not remove your gloves until you have disposed of all sharps and clinical waste
- If you have to remove your gloves (e.g. after a per rectum exam), put on new non-sterile gloves before you continue disposing of clinical waste
- Mentally check that all the sharps you unwrapped have been accounted for

---

OSCE Key Learning Points

✔ Ensure you have the appropriate equipment, sharps bin, and waste bag within reach

✔ Put on personal protective equipment: gloves and apron are a minimum

✔ Dispose of sharps directly after using them: do not put them down anywhere

✔ Dispose of clinical waste straight into a yellow bag: do not let it touch any other surfaces

✔ Remove your gloves only when all waste has been disposed of

---

Complications

Needle-stick injuries

- A 'needle-stick' is a injury caused by a contaminated sharp (i.e. one which has been in contact with a patient)
- Gloves reduce the likelihood of a blood-borne virus being transmitted by needle-stick: they 'clean' the needle as it travels through the material of the glove
- If you receive a needle-stick, clean away your sharps and clinical waste, and then wash the wound under running water. Let it bleed, but do not squeeze it (local inflammation increases the risk of HIV transmission)
- Alert your team to what has happened. Within working hours, call your occupational health department for advice. Out of hours, go to A&E for advice
- Often you will be advised to find out if the patient would be willing to be tested for HIV and viral hepatitis. You must ask a colleague to approach the patient after a needle-stick injury, as you have a vested interest in the patient getting tested

- If the patient is known to have HIV, or is 'high risk' (e.g. an intravenous drug user or a sex worker), you may be offered post-exposure prophylaxis. This is a course of antiretrovirals that reduces your risk of developing HIV after exposure. It is most effective if started within 24 hours of a needle-stick. Occupational health and A&E will be able to provide this, if appropriate

Splash injuries

- A splash injury is when a patient's bodily fluids (e.g. blood, amniotic fluid, faeces) touch your mucus membranes or eyes
- Splash injuries can be avoided by use of appropriate personal protective equipment
- If you think you may have received a splash injury, contact your occupational health department for advice

'Clean' sharps injuries

- If you cut yourself on a sharp that has not been in contact with a patient (e.g. a broken glass ampoule or a clean scalpel blade), there is no need to contact occupational health, unless the injury is severe enough to affect your work or study
- Follow the usual first aid protocols for cuts. Ask someone to help you clean and dress your wound, using appropriate protocols. Do not make a mess
- Remember that your blood is clinical waste too!

 Common misinterpretations and pitfalls

- Splash injuries are dangerous too
- Sharps injuries are common, but most are avoidable

33 Arterial blood gas sampling

Introduction

Arterial blood gas (ABG) samples provide an aid to diagnosis in a multitude of conditions. The most important values are:

- pH
- Arterial oxygen values
- Arterial carbon dioxide values
- Bicarbonate
- Lactate
- Electrolytes

Indications

ABG sampling is indicated in variety of clinical settings, including:

- Respiratory failure type 1 and 2
- Diabetic ketoacidosis
- Severe renal failure
- Drug overdose
- Sepsis
- Post cardiac arrest

 NB ABG sampling is helpful with the diagnosis and management of many conditions.

Cautions

- Some people find this procedure uncomfortable and patients should be warned of this. Local anaesthetic can be used if required

Medical Student Survival Skills: Procedural Skills, First Edition. Philip Jevon and Ruchi Joshi.
© 2020 John Wiley & Sons Ltd. Published 2020 by John Wiley & Sons Ltd.
Companion website: www.wiley.com/go/jevon/medicalstudent

- Allen's test should be completed before beginning the procedure as there is a risk of damaging the artery
- Always use a heparinised syringe to take the sample to prevent coagulation of sample

Allen's test

- Ask the patient to clench their fist (if they are unable to do so, tightly close their hand)
- Apply occlusive pressure, using the fingers, to the ulnar and radial arteries (to obstruct blood flow to the hand)
- While applying this pressure, ask the patient to relax their hand; observe the palm and fingers for blanching (this will confirm occlusion of both arteries)
- Release the occlusive pressure from the ulnar artery; this will confirm whether the modified Allen's test is positive or negative

---

OSCE Key Learning Points

Allen's test

✔ *Positive Allen's test:* hand flushes within 5–15 seconds indicating adequate perfusion through the ulnar artery
✔ *Negative Allen's test:* hand does not flush within 5–15 seconds indicating inadequate perfusion through the ulnar artery, i.e. the radial artery in that hand should not be punctured

---

Contraindications

- Abnormal Allen's test
- Damaged vessel
- Infection over arterial site
- Site of arteriovenous fistula
- Coagulopathy – relative contraindication

Equipment

- ChloraPrep (or other cleaning solution)
- Non-sterile gloves

- 22G needle
- Heparinised ABG syringe
- Gauze
- Fixation tape

Procedure for insertion

Pre-procedure

- Prepare equipment:
- Identify correct patient – name, date of birth
- Explain procedure to the patient and obtain consent
- Warn the patient of pain and ask them to remain as still as possible
- Complete Allen's test
- Wash hands and don non-sterile gloves

Procedure

- Position patient's hand appropriately with wrist slightly extended
- Select site of arterial puncture – the radial is most commonly used (other possible sites include brachial and femoral)
- Palpate the artery and find the area of maximal pulsation. The radial artery can be felt from the base of the thumb to the mid forearm
- Clean the area with cleaning equipment
- Keep your non-dominant index finger on the arterial pulsation throughout
- Hold the needle and syringe like a dart
- At the place of maximal pulsation insert the needle at an angle of 45° towards the artery with the needles bevel facing up
- Blood will flash back into the syringe without aspiration
- Hold the needle steady whilst the syringe fills. You may need to pull back on the plunger
- Once you have an adequate sample (normally 1–3 ml), withdraw the needle
- Apply firm pressure over the site with gauze for a minimum of 2 minutes.

Post-procedure

- Apply fixation tape over the gauze to maintain pressure on the area
- Apply pressure to the site to reduce the risk of haematoma formation
- Discard all sharps and rubbish appropriately
- Expel excess air from the sample and place a cap on the syringe

- Immediately take the arterial blood sample to a gas analyser whilst agitating the sample
- Ensure you make a note of the patient's current oxygen support as this allows more accurate interpretation of results

OSCE Key Learning Points

- Find site of maximal palpation – take your time!
- If you get no flashback, pull back the needle and readvance at a slightly different angle
- Ensure pressure is applied post-procedure

Complications

- Pain over site
- Active bleeding from site
- Haematoma
- Infection
- Ischaemia distal to the vessel

 Common misinterpretations and pitfalls

ABG sampling can be difficult to interpret. Read around this topic so you are familiar with the normal values and what abnormal results suggest.

34 Examination of the ear

Introduction

Examination of the ear is a very important, especially in the young.

- Children often present with ear problems ranging from foreign bodies to infections
- Ear examination is very important in very young children with a fever
- Examining the ear requires much practice to help appreciate what is normal from abnormal

Otological symptoms

Patients may present with any of the following symptoms:

- Otalgia – pain originating from inside the ear, the pinna. Some conditions may produce pain referred to the ear
- Otorrhoea – discharge from the ear
- Tinnitus – a ringing sensation in the ear not from an external stimulus
- Vertigo – a sensation of the room spinning and loss of balance
- Hearing loss

Conditions encountered on examination

External ear

- Infection – perichondritis, cellulitis
- Trauma to the pinna – haematoma, laceration
- Carcinoma – basal or squamous cell carcinoma, malignant melanoma
- Congenital malformations
- Mastoiditis

Medical Student Survival Skills: Procedural Skills, First Edition. Philip Jevon and Ruchi Joshi.
© 2020 John Wiley & Sons Ltd. Published 2020 by John Wiley & Sons Ltd.
Companion website: www.wiley.com/go/jevon/medicalstudent

External auditory canal

- Infection – otitis externa, malignant otitis externa, folliculitis/abscess, herpes zoster infection
- Systemic skin conditions – eczema, seborrhoeic dermatitis
- Wax impaction
- Foreign body

Tympanic membrane

- Tympanic membrane perforation/retraction pocket
- Tympanosclerosis
- Cholesteatoma
- Grommet/ventilation tube

Middle ear

- Acute suppurative otitis media
- Otitis media with effusion (glue ear)
- Chronic suppurative otitis media
- Ossicular pathology – difficult to assess with simple examination

Inner ear

- Inner ear conditions are difficult to assess with simple examination techniques and usually require detailed imaging and hearing tests.

Indications

Examine the ears in anyone presenting with the above otological symptoms or in any restless child with a fever.

 NB Always examine ears in pyrexic, restless children.

Cautions

- Examination of the ear in children can be a frightening experience, so you must be very gentle and get help from a parent or carer
- Infection of the ear canal is usually very painful so care must be taken when introducing the otoscope

Equipment

- Otoscope
- Correct sized otoscope cap
- Non-sterile gloves

Procedure

Pre-procedure

- Prepare equipment
- Identify correct patient
- Obtain consent from patient
- Explain procedure to the patient
- Wash hands and don non-sterile gloves

Procedure

- Inspect the pinna and outer ear from the side – looking for swelling, erythema, scars, deformity and any discharge from the canal
- Move the pinna forward, looking behind the ear, examing for postauricular scar and mastoid swelling
- Palpate the mastoid process for tenderness
- Use one hand to straighten the ear canal by pulling the pinna:
  - Adults – superior and posteriorly
  - Children – inferior and posteriorly
- Hold the otosocope in the same hand to the side you are examining, holding it like a pen. Keep the little finger free and against the side of the patient's head for security
- As you insert the otosocope inspect all four walls of the external canal (Figure 34.1)
- Examine the tympanic membrane:
  - Identify the handle of the malleus and the light reflex
  - Inspect the tympanic membrane in all four quadrants
  - Remember to look at the superior part of the membrane (attic) for any evidence of cholesteatoma
- Remove the otosocope after successful examination
- To complete the examination you can assess hearing with speech:
  - At a distance of 60 cm from each ear firstly whisper, then talk normally, and then loudly

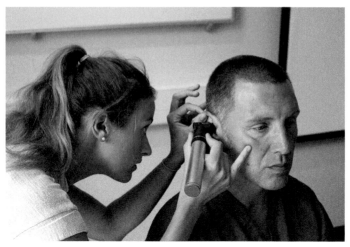

Figure 34.1 Examination of the ear.

- Bisyllabic words can be used
- The contralateral ear should be masked
- Tuning fork test can also be used to assess hearing:
  - Use a 256 or 512 Hz tuning fork
  - Perform Rinne's test and Weber's test to identify any conductive or sensorineural hearing loss
  - Rinne's test:
    - Air conduction is louder than bone conduction
    - Strike the tuning fork and hold 2 cm away from the ear for air conduction
    - Then hold it against the mastoid process for bone conduction
    - Ask the patient which was louder
    - In normal hearing air conduction is louder – Rinne's test is positive (however this could also suggest sensorinerual hearing loss on the same side)
    - Rinne's test is negative – bone conduction is louder than air conduction indicating conductive hearing loss on that side
  - Weber's test:
    - The tuning fork is held on the vertex
    - With normal hearing the sound is localised to the vertex
    - In conductive deafness the sound is localised to the affected ear
    - In sensorineural deafness the sound is localised to the unaffected ear

Post-procedure

- To complete the examination you should examine the oropharynx and the neck
- Thank the patient and wash your hands

OSCE Key Learning Points

 Always remember to examine behind the ears

Carefully introduce the otoscope into the ear

Remember to inspect all four quadrants of the tympanic membrane including the attic

Complications

- Very few complications can arise – it is generally a safe examination

⚠ Common misinterpretations and pitfalls

- Otological symptoms can be referred – thus the nose and throat should form part of the complete examination
- Only middle ear and external ear conditions are visible on examination of the ear

35 Ophthalmoscopy

Introduction

- Ophthalmoscopy (fundoscopy) is performed to examine the eye
- It is predominantly used to examine the retina, but can also be used to examine the cornea and lens of the eye
- It is only one component of a general eye examination

Ophthalmological problems

Direct ophthalmoscopy can be used to identify a range of problems with the eye.

Abnormal red reflex

If a red reflex is present it means that light shone into the eyes is reflected back from the retina. If it is absent it means that the light is obstructed at some point along this path.

Common causes of an abnormal red reflex include:

- Congenital – corneal opacities, cataract, glaucoma, vitreous opacities, retinoblastoma
- Corneal scarring or infection
- Anterior chamber
  - Bleeding (hyphaema) – blood accumulates in the anterior chamber, e.g. after trauma
  - Infection/inflammation – white cells accumulate in the anterior chamber (hypopyon)
- Lens
  - Cataract
- Posterior chamber
  - Vitreous haemorrhage

Medical Student Survival Skills: Procedural Skills, First Edition. Philip Jevon and Ruchi Joshi.
© 2020 John Wiley & Sons Ltd. Published 2020 by John Wiley & Sons Ltd.
Companion website: www.wiley.com/go/jevon/medicalstudent

- Retina
  - Retinal detachment
  - Tumour, e.g. melanoma

Abnormal optic disc

- Optic disc swelling (papilloedema) occurs in conditions where the neurons are damaged (either within the eye or along their course into the brain). Damage can be caused by:
- Trauma, e.g. compression of the nerve in patients with raised intracranial pressure
- Inflammation, e.g. optic neuritis in multiple sclerosis
- Ischaemia, e.g. central retinal vein occlusion, vasculitis
- Toxins, e.g. toxic optic neuropathy in methanol poisoning
- Idiopathic, e.g. idiopathic intracranial hypertension (previously known as benign intracranial hypertension)

  Optic disc atrophy occurs where neurons die completely. The thickness of the rim of the optic disc is reduced (greater cup to disc ratio). Glaucoma is the most common condition associated with this but any disease that damages the neurons will also cause optic atrophy.

Abnormal retina

- Swelling is difficult to assess on fundoscopy because there is no three-dimensional view. Common causes include:
  - Drusen – yellow deposits of material which are a normal feature of advancing age. They are also associated with age-related macular degeneration (AMD)
  - Fluid, e.g. macular oedema
- White scar tissue
  - Scarring may be a signs of a previous infection, e.g. cytomegalovirus retinitis
  - It also occurs after laser treatment for retinal detachment or diabetic retinopathy
- Pigment deposits are seen as star-shaped black deposits on the retina, also known as bone spicules. In retinitis pigmentosa many of these are seen around the edge of the retina
- Abnormal blood vessels (microaneurysms, abnormal tortuous new vessels) and the consequence of abnormal new vessels (flame haemorrhage, cotton wool spots, hard exudates) – these are seen in diabetic retinopathy

Indications

- Concern about eye problem, e.g. increasingly blurred vision
- Concern about raised intracranial pressure, e.g. headaches
- Monitoring systemic disease, e.g. diabetes
- Red reflex assessed as part of newborn screening examination

Contraindications

- Patient refusal

Equipment

- Ophthalmoscope

Procedure for examination

Preparation

- Wash hands
- Identify correct patient
- Introduce yourself
- Explain procedure briefly and gain consent
- Consider administering dilating drops (1% tropicamide)
  - Check visual acuity before dilating pupils!
  - Dilating drops are contraindicated if the patient has an allergy to tropicamide, is driving, or an urgent referral to the ophthalmologist is likely as they limit the ophthalmologist's ability to examine the eye
- Set up the ophthalmoscope
  - Select a medium or small aperture if undilated, and a large aperture if dilated
  - Set the focusing wheel to 0 if you do not wear glasses or are wearing glasses. Alternatively take your glasses off and set the focusing wheel to your prescription
- Darken the room

Procedure

- Ask the patient to fix on a point in the distance, e.g. a small feature on a poster on a wall behind you
- Warn the patient that you will come very close to their face in order to get the best view possible

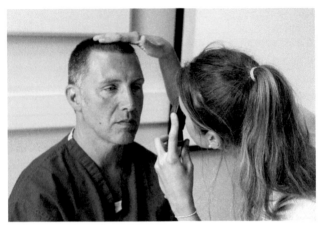

Figure 35.1 Ophthalmoscopy: correct positioning.

- If you are examining the patient's right eye, hold the ophthalmoscope to your right eye with your right hand, and vice versa for the left eye
- Place your free hand on the patient's forehead (Figure 35.1)
- Hold the ophthalmoscope to your eye. Rest it on your eyebrow or cheek and fix it here. From now on, the head and ophthalmoscope move as one
- Shine the light into the pupil of the eye being examined. It should reflect back brightly, this is known as the red reflex
- Come close to the eye, always following the red reflex. If you lose the red reflex, simply come back and re-centre and then approach the patient again
- Once you are as close as possible to the patient (as close as a centimetre from the patient's face), while still focusing on the red reflex, adjust the focusing wheel until the retinal vessels are clear. In a patient with 20:20 vision little adjustment is required
- Follow the path of the retinal vessels to the optic disc
- Examine the optic disc for swelling and cup to disc ratio. The cup to disc ratio compares the diameter of the cup to the diameter of the disc. A large ratio suggests optic disc atrophy
- Follow the path of each of the four main ophthalmic vessels (superior temporal, superior nasal, inferior nasal, inferior temporal), examining the surrounding retina and blood vessels as you do so
- Examine the fundus and macula by asking the patient to 'look into the light'

Post-procedure

- Thank the patient
- Wash your hands
- Summarise your findings and document

OSCE Key Learning Points

✔ Dim the lights and ask the patient to focus on a distant point

✔ Set the dial to a medium aperture, focusing the wheel to 0

✔ Find the red reflex and follow it

✔ Three key abnormalities to look for include: (i) abnormal red reflex, (ii) a swollen or atrophic optic disc, and (iii) retinal scarring, pigment deposits, or abnormal blood vessels

✔ Key diseases that can come up in the OSCE are cataract, papilloedema, photocoagulation laser, retinitis pigmentosa, and diabetic retinopathy

36 Relieving foreign body airway obstruction

Introduction

- Foreign body airway obstruction (FBAO) (choking) is a life-threatening emergency
- An uncommon but potentially treatable cause of accidental death, it is usually associated with eating and is therefore commonly witnessed
- Prompt recognition and effective intervention are paramount

Signs

Signs of FBAO will depend upon whether it is partial or complete.

- *Partial airway obstruction*: the patient will be distressed, may cough, and may be wheezy
- *Complete airway obstruction*: the patient is unable to talk, unable to breathe or cough, and has maximal respiratory effort, development of cyanosis, and clutching of the neck; the patient will be very distressed

 NB FBAO is often associated with eating and is usually witnessed.

Procedure

- Ask the patient 'are you choking?' If they are choking, but able to breathe and talk, encourage them to cough. However, if they are choking and unable to breathe and talk (may say 'yes' by nodding the head without speaking), this indicates severe airway obstruction requiring urgent treatment
- Stand at their side, slightly behind them

Medical Student Survival Skills: Procedural Skills, First Edition. Philip Jevon and Ruchi Joshi.
© 2020 John Wiley & Sons Ltd. Published 2020 by John Wiley & Sons Ltd.
Companion website: www.wiley.com/go/jevon/medicalstudent

- Lean the patient forward. This will help ensure that, if the foreign body is dislodged, it drops out of the mouth instead of slipping further down the airway. If appropriate, support their chest using one hand
- Deliver up to five back blows between the scapulas using the heel of the hand (Figure 36.1), checking after each one if the FBAO has been relieved. If the back blows fail, deliver abdominal thrusts
- Stand behind the patient and encircle the upper abdomen with your arms
- Lean the patient forward and place a clenched fist between their umbilicus and xiphisternum and clasp it with the other hand (Figure 36.2)
- Deliver up to five abdominal thrusts, checking after each one if the FBAO has been relieved
- If FBAO remains, continue alternating five back blows with five abdominal thrusts
- If the patient loses consciousness, carefully support them to the floor and start cardiopulmonary resuscitation (it is possible that chest compressions may relieve the FBAO)
- Ensure someone has called 999 for an ambulance

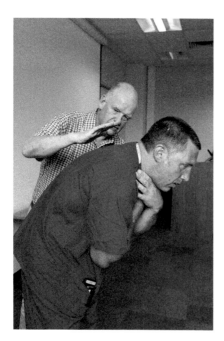

Figure 36.1 Back slaps.

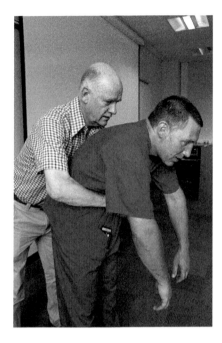

Figure 36.2 Abdominal thrusts.

Follow-up management

- If measures are successful at relieving FBAO, it is still possible that the foreign body could be lodged in the airways: therefore if the victim has dysphagia, persistent cough, or complains of having something 'stuck in his throat', they should be referred to a doctor
- If abdominal thrusts were performed, advise the victim to see a doctor because serious internal injury (e.g. rupture or laceration of abdominal or thoracic viscera) may have been caused

Index

Note: Page numbers in *italics* refer to figures.
Page numbers in **bold** refer to tables.

Medical Student Survival Skills: Procedural Skills, First Edition. Philip Jevon and Ruchi Joshi.
© 2020 John Wiley & Sons Ltd. Published 2020 by John Wiley & Sons Ltd.
Companion website: www.wiley.com/go/jevon/medicalstudent